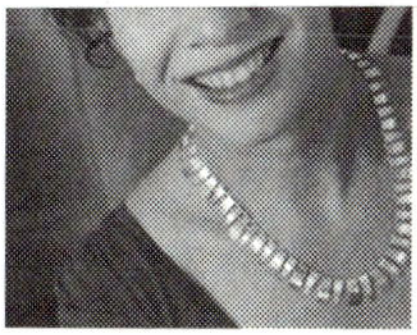

Sally Collings is the author of 2007 bestseller *Sophie's Journey*. Sally worked in book publishing for almost 20 years, dividing her time between London and Sydney. Now based in Brisbane and a mother of two, she is a freelance writer and editor, specialising in life stories and inspirational writing of all kinds.

Wishing you well -

Sally Collings

Positive

finding life in the midst of cancer

Sally Collings

HarperCollins*Publishers*

HarperCollins*Publishers*

First published in Australia in 2009
by HarperCollins*Publishers* Australia Pty Limited
ABN 36 009 913 517
www.harpercollins.com.au

HarperCollins*Publishers*
25 Ryde Road, Pymble, Sydney, NSW 2073, Australia
31 View Road, Glenfield, Auckland 0627, New Zealand
1–A, Hamilton House, Connaught Place, New Delhi – 110 001, India
77–85 Fulham Palace Road, London, W6 8JB, United Kingdom
2 Bloor Street East, 20th floor, Toronto, Ontario M4W 1A8, Canada
10 East 53rd Street, New York NY 10022, USA

National Library of Australia Cataloguing-in-Publication data:

Collings, Sally.
Positive : finding life in the midst of cancer / Sally Collings.
ISBN: 978 07322 8719 1 (pbk.)
Cancer – Patients – Personal narratives.
Cancer – Patients – Anecdotes.
Cancer – Anecdotes.
Cancer – Patients – Information services.
Cancer – Patients – Life skills guides.
362.19699400922

Cover image by imageworks/Getty Images
Cover design by Darren Holt, HarperCollins Design Studio
Typeset in 11.5/17 Bembo by Kirby Jones
Printed and bound in Australia by Griffin Press
70gsm Classic used by HarperCollins*Publishers* is a natural, recyclable product made from wood grown in sustainable forests. The manufacturing processes conform to the environmental regulations in the country of origin, Finland.

5 4 3 2 1 09 10 11 12

For Valerie Elisabeth Harper (1928–2003)

'Death is not extinguishing the light; it is only putting out the lamp because the dawn has come.'

Rabindranath Tagore (1861–1941)

Contents

Introduction

Positive. It may be a diagnosis, an outcome, an attitude or a relationship. The term describes the 'upside' of cancer that appears against all expectations and, seemingly, against the odds.

The positives are not immediate, or apparent all the time, or there for everyone. Sometimes the benefits aren't visible until years later. And as the stories in this book show, sometimes they are not even for you but for your brother, wife, daughter, friend.

This book represents a collection of voices: cancer survivors, carers, husbands, parents, sisters. Together, their stories map out the terrain of the upside of cancer: the opportunity to draw together (as friends, as a couple, as a family); the torrent of support, love and prayers that are unleashed; and the impetus to go deeper and embrace the strength, fears and purpose that lie within each of us.

When I started to write *Positive*, I could see no good in cancer. My mother died of lung cancer in 2003, and I found find no positives in that. If I tried hard I was able to convince myself that it could have been worse. Mum died just four months after her diagnosis, and she was cared for at home until the final days of her life. She didn't want any long, drawn-out treatment postponing the inevitable, so in a way she had the end that she would have wished for.

My mother died one week after my first daughter, Bethany, was born. She had been over the moon about my pregnancy, though in her typically understated way; anyone less close to her might not have noticed. By the time of Bethany's birth at the end of June, Mum was pretty much confined to bed. Still, I could tell by the gleam in her eyes she was pleased to see me with my new baby, although by then everything was an effort — breathing most of all. It was terrible to see my clever, observant mother reduced to struggling for each breath. Yet she lived to see my baby girl, her granddaughter. Born to her roaming restless daughter, who was then in her late thirties; it was a blessing that my mother had perhaps long since ceased to wish for.

Mum was a heavy smoker for about 40 years; I remember her sitting in her favourite chair in the living room, reading the latest crime novel from the local library, shrouded in a haze of grey smoke lit by the bars of light coming through the venetian blinds. She amazed us all by giving up smoking late in life — too late to repair the damage. Although she died soon after her cancer diagnosis, you could equally say she was dying from the time she smoked her first cigarette. So I expected Mum's death, but that didn't make it any easier. Expectation comes from the head, but grief is a thing of the heart, quite unrelated. At least they say it's in the heart, but to me it felt like a well of sorrow at the bottom of my stomach that would fill up from time to time. I could clearly feel the level of sadness rising then, lapping at my ribs, my chest, right up to the base of my throat.

I could see no true positives. Saying 'it could have been worse' was just making the best out of a tragic situation. That didn't make it good. Then one day, four years after my mother died, I read an article which said that nearly two out of three cancer survivors and their families consider that something good has come out of their experience.* I could see on an intellectual level that benefits could occur through cancer, and I was moved to know that it happened for others, even though that wasn't my story. All the same, I was intrigued that the majority of people could see some upside to cancer, and I had a feeling that in that concept, there was a remarkable book waiting to be written. That vague feeling turned to an insistent urge, and the idea for *Positive* was born. Even so, the connection with my own situation was buried so deep in my psyche that I was a full month into the project before I realised how personal this book would be for me.

---

* *USA Today*/Kaiser Family Foundation/Harvard School of Public Health Cancer Survey (conducted 1 August–14 September 2006)

You won't find a lot of advice in these pages. Many of the people whose stories appear here were wary of offering guidance; their journey was such a personal one, they were reluctant to offer any words of wisdom for others. Instead, this is a book of reflection and possibilities.

In the course of writing *Positive,* I spoke to hundreds of people about their own stories and stories they had heard: cancer support workers, hospital staff, advocates, counsellors, survivors, carers, relatives, friends — including those who would soon lose their own lives to cancer. Over and over again, the people I spoke with welcomed the idea of the book, and the potential it had to offer hope and shared experiences. I expected it to be a hard sell — to explain what I meant by 'positive' and to find people who identified with that experience and were willing to share their stories in print. It wasn't.

Some people did react angrily to the idea behind this book. One teenage boy whose uncle had died of cancer a year before was explosively hostile: 'The whole idea is trite! How can you say that anything good comes out of someone dying?' Or the grieving mother with young children whose husband died from a brain tumour: 'I lost my husband, my two daughters lost their father — what's positive about that?'

They were rare exceptions, though — surprisingly rare, given the immeasurable cost of cancer in the currency of grief and pain. Most people I spoke to understood the idea immediately, and I had far more offers of stories than I could possibly do justice to in a single volume. People generously gave their time and their personal accounts, digging deep to reflect on the part cancer had played in their lives in the hope that their stories would speak into the hearts of those on a parallel path.

As I talked to all these people, I came to realise that for me, my 'positive' is this book. Creating it enabled me to find other ways of perceiving my own experience, and it allowed me to do something that might inspire other people. I hope that you will read *Positive* and find in it a story that strikes a chord of hope for you, or convinces you to keep going, or to make something good out of an otherwise tragic circumstance. Then my positive will become yours.

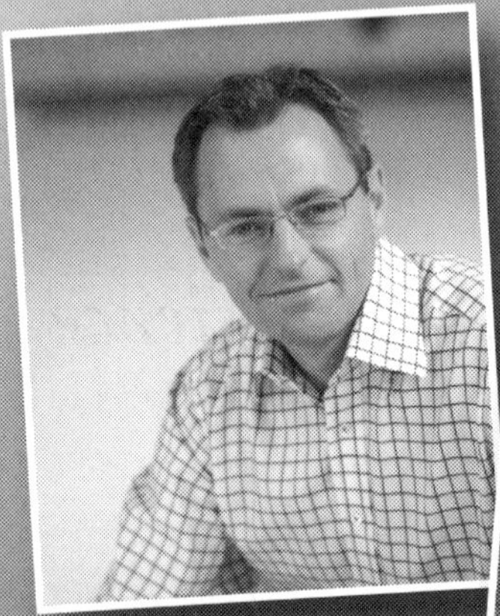
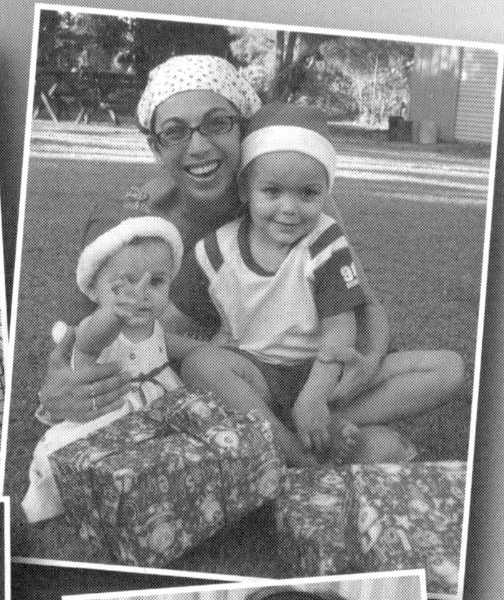
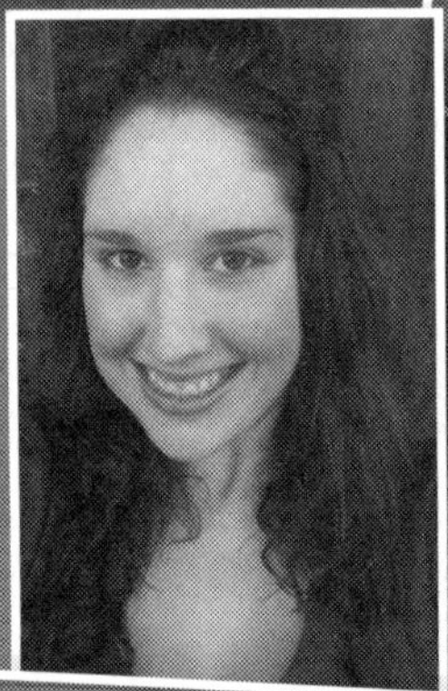
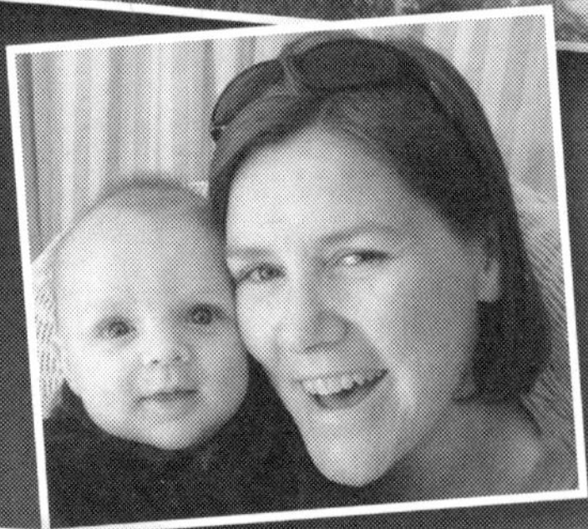
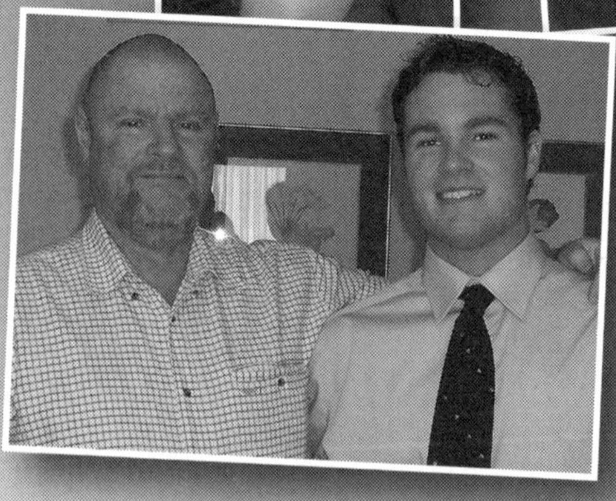
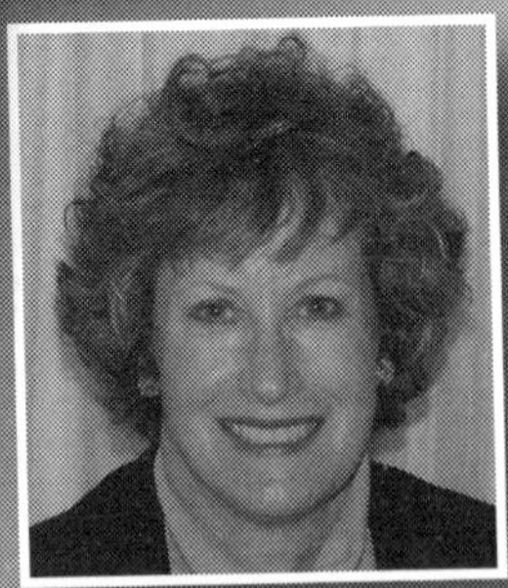

CHAPTER 1

A mind-altering experience

> Just as a game, tell yourself that you could be six weeks from the end of your life. Right now. You could be! Suddenly a lot of complicated things become very simple. You can forget about all the things that revolve around you, and start focusing on the reasons you were given this life in the first place. Find what it is that binds you to this life, because we're given the opportunity to work on that every single day. And then one day, suddenly, it can all be taken away.
>
> **Pianist Aaron McMillan on *Australian Story* in September 2001 (Aaron died in May 2007)**

When someone starts walking the cancer path, the changes start in their body even before their mind is aware of it. But from the instant the word 'cancer' is uttered in the doctor's surgery, people's thoughts are racing, trying to catch all of the implications, outcomes, impacts, possibilities.

In the face of a cancer diagnosis there is a prevailing sequence of responses. It is essentially a process of grief:

denial and numbness are overtaken by anger, which gives way to sadness (and often depression) before acceptance can make an appearance at last.

Further down the track, it's possible for some people to talk about lessons learned in the 'cancer classroom'. It seems a unanimous verdict that they wouldn't wish that particular course of study on anyone, friend or enemy, but neither would they have gained certain insights without attending those classes themselves.

At the same time, the idea that your attitude can dictate your health — mind over matter — is both a touchstone of hope and an enormous source of guilt among cancer patients. If you have a positive outlook, some people say, you can beat cancer. But by implication, if cancer beats you, maybe you weren't positive enough. Sometimes there is a touch of magical thinking going on here, as psychologist Dr Jane Turner suggests on page 24 — a superstitious belief that 'if I behave like this or stop doing that, the cancer will go away'.

Some of the people who appear in this section do believe strongly in the power of the mind and the individual's ability to overcome cancer. It all depends on what you mean by 'overcoming': for people like Jason Garrick (page 42), if you succumb to negativity, you've lost the battle. It's not a question of physical healing: the bigger triumph may be new insights, attitudes, perspectives. And the new challenge may be hanging on to that view of the world long after the chemotherapy has finished.

Chris Reason

All of a sudden there was this intriguing moment — an epiphany of sorts — when I thought, 'My existence has suddenly come down to two extremes: life and death.' Everything else in between didn't matter any more. The clothes, the bills, ambitions, possessions — all of those things became absolutely irrelevant. The paramount thing in my existence at the time was to survive. Suddenly life became very black and white, and it was a wonderful feeling.

Television reporter and presenter Chris Reason has seen more dangerous situations than most: the Bosnian War, the Kobe earthquake, the Thredbo landslide. He is also a survivor of testicular cancer. Originally diagnosed in 1998, Chris had a yearly check each September. Then in 2001 he was sent to cover the attacks on the World Trade Center, and his annual check-up slipped his mind. A year later, when he remembered, the test revealed that a Stage 2 cancer had reached his kidneys and lymphatic system. In the course of his treatment, everything Chris once considered important was stripped away: his job, his relationship, his health. Now married and clear of cancer, in 2007 Chris and his wife, Kathryn Robinson, became the parents of twins.

CHRIS REASON: When I was first diagnosed, everything in my life stopped. There are few more terrifying words in the

English language than 'cancer'. Perhaps only 'chemotherapy' tops it. When you get both words delivered in a sentence by your doctor, the effect is devastating. But I went on to learn valuable life lessons both times I went through my cancer battles. I came out of the experience a very different person, a better person.

The first time around, in those initial months after being discharged from hospital, my cancer experiences shaped who I was and how I viewed the world. But to be honest, the lessons I learned started to slip from the memory as time went by and the impact of the cancer experience started to fade. The challenge I give myself is to not let that happen — to try and hold on to those memories, the lessons learned, the promises I made myself. I try to constantly remind myself of the perspective cancer survival gave me. Whatever is happening to me — a bad day at work, a fight with my wife — I try and stop myself and think, 'Put all this back in perspective, Chris, and remember the black hole you were in back in 2002.' I guess that is the overall impact that surviving cancer has had for me — it gives me a deep and profound appreciation for the life that I have and the health that I have; the challenge is to never let myself forget that.

I was a pretty dumb cancer patient. I initially ignored all the telltale signs that something was wrong with my 'man parts'. Despite my right testicle being almost twice the size of the left, I just ignored it, foolishly thinking that any growth in that part of the male anatomy was a good thing

— and that perhaps the other parts would follow suit! I let it go for six months before I went to see a doctor. A stupid, stupid decision that almost cost me my life. That was 1998, when I was first diagnosed with testicular cancer. Well, I survived that, but then, in another display of male stupidity, I missed my annual check-up three years later because I let my career get in the way. I raced off to the United States to cover the September 11 attacks and didn't even think about the check-up until the following year. By then it was too late; the cancer had spread through the lymphatic system to the kidneys and I needed treatment: six months of operations and chemotherapy. So, one of the major promises I've made to myself is never to be so complacent again.

There are dozens of other promises I made myself after that battle: 'I promise to eat better, eat organic, not stress so much, work hard for cancer charities, exercise more ...' Lists of them. But they're like New Year's resolutions: hard to keep going past 31 January. If I could nominate the most important one, it is this: I promise not to forget the glimpse I was given of what life is all about. It came at about the three-quarter mark in my battle, the lowest of the low points. Everything was going wrong for me. The chemo wasn't working, the tumours weren't going. I'd lost so much weight, I'd lost all the hair on my body, lost the job I'd spent a career trying to get, lost my girlfriend — everything just came crashing down.

But all of a sudden there was this intriguing moment — an epiphany of sorts — when I thought, 'My existence has suddenly come down to two extremes: life and death.' Everything else in between didn't matter any more. The clothes, the bills, ambitions, possessions — all of those things became absolutely irrelevant. The paramount thing in my existence at the time was to survive. There is something extremely liberating about that; it was almost religious, spiritual. Suddenly life became very black and white, and it was a wonderful feeling. The stress of my situation disappeared, the goal posts suddenly appeared from the mists, and I knew what direction I needed to head in. I'm convinced it was a turning point for me; it really helped carry me through.

One of my operations left a huge scar down my abdomen. Every day when I get out of the shower, I see it in the mirror and I try and use it to remind myself of that state of mind I was in mid-battle. It just puts the chaos of the day into very sharp perspective. That's my most important promise to myself — not to forget that lesson from the cancer classroom.

Support was paramount during the darker times — and often came as a surprise as well. I was hosting a TV show at the time, *Sunrise*. We'd just started the show; it was nine months old when I got my diagnosis and I had to leave the program. I was amazed by how many people contacted me, wrote letters and cards and sent get-well presents, just to let me know they were thinking of me and that I'd touched their lives in some way. It was a phenomenal feeling, to have that extra support beyond the family, beyond the friendship circles

— literally thousands of strangers out there had taken the time to write in. Of course family support was extraordinarily important. I wasn't married at the time, and my family basically came to my side; they all lived interstate and they all drove in or flew down. Week after week they took turns to drive me back and forth to hospital and do the cleaning and cooking and all those things. They moved into my flat and just lived with me; that got me through. Friends did as well; many were dropping over meals, offering advice and support — that was amazing. A lot of people gave me books and various methods and suggestions for battling cancer. You can't take all of it in, but there was one that struck a chord: Dr Ian Gawler's book, *You Can Conquer Cancer.* I carried it everywhere, I read it a dozen times during my cancer and found it an extremely practical tool to help back up what I myself was doing and what my doctors were doing for me.

The oncology nurses at Royal North Shore Hospital were unbelievable, too; they were at my side all the time, and at the darkest moments. At the three- or four-month mark, the weight of it just came crashing down on me; some random day, when the nurse was queuing up to stick another needle in my arm for another five or six hours of chemo, I burst into tears. I just lost it, sitting in the chemo ward. They were fantastic; they swung into action, got me a counsellor. For the first time in my life I saw a psychologist, and in an hour-long session I poured out everything I'd been bottling up: all the bravery, all the false positives, all of the attitude that you are expected to take with you in a medical battle like that. The nurses gave me something that I would never have done by myself: I would never have picked up the phone and rung a psychologist or psychiatrist.

Wednesday 5 March 2003 was the end of the battle. The doctors were extremely confident when they let me leave hospital. They said, 'We don't often use the word cured, but we think you are cured. You are not in remission — it's over.' Once a year I go and have the tests to check, and there is a tension a couple of weeks before the CAT scans and blood tests. You do think, 'What if it is back, is there a chance, why is my lower back a little bit painful, what does this mean?' So it never does go away; it is always lingering, sitting on the shoulder. I reached the five-year mark last March, which was an important one; they say five years out from testicular cancer is pretty much the all-clear. There was no signs of any recurrence, so it doesn't get much better than that. But beyond that — I still think that the tension will be there, but I don't bow to it that much. I genuinely believe that I have it beat.

I just think myself so lucky to have got to this position: not only to survive the disease, but two weeks after 5 March, I met Kath for the first time, and she later went on to become my wife. Four years down the track, we had twins. It's so uplifting, to have something as wonderful as the twins come along. When we were pregnant, we were at the hospital where I'd been battling for my life four years earlier. When we got the news that it was twins we took the elevator downstairs and I said to Kath, 'Let's just duck in here and say hello to Polly and the girls and let them know the news.' We walked in there and we told them, and there were tears; it was a terrific moment.

I feel a lot braver about death now. It is something you have to confront; I don't think you can ignore it, I don't think it's healthy or wise to. I can honestly say I accepted [the possibility of my] death; I was certainly not happy enough to let it happen, but I was prepared to accept it. I'd had an extraordinary life up until that time and I'd achieved most of the things I'd wanted to — in my career, in my life, in my travels, in everything I set myself. The only thing I was lacking at that stage was family, my own family, and I wanted that badly. But I think I was as prepared as I could be for death.

If nothing else, [cancer] forces you to confront all those core issues of life and death. You have to think about the big picture; after several months of battle, the minutiae finally get swept away and it just comes down to the bare basics of life — your health, your life, will you die, relationships, what's got to be patched up, what's got to be nurtured more. In a funny way, it is one of the benefits that you get from struggling through cancer. It's not all doom and gloom, it's not all bleak; you can extract many things from your fight. It shows you what you are made of, it shows you how you react under the greatest duress and the greatest pressures life can throw at you. You learn a lot from cancer; it can be a very ugly thing, but a very moving, positive experience in so many ways.

Bernadette Vella

Strangely enough, I actually feel ready to die, with one exception: I need to be a mum to my kids for a lot longer — they are not ready to lose me yet, and my job with them is not finished … Maybe one day, when they are all grown up, the cancer will come back and I will not be able to fight it, but until that stage if it does come back, it is not winning, because God help anything that tries to come between me and my kids.

Bernadette was just 14 weeks pregnant with her second child when she was diagnosed with Hodgkin's lymphoma. She had had trouble breathing and went to the emergency department of her local hospital. Immediately she was faced with the sort of decision every pregnant woman dreads: should she go through the full barrage of treatment, or would the risk to her unborn child be too much? Bernadette decided to have treatment in the hope that she would be there to see her children grow up. The gamble paid off: her daughter, Arielle, was born premature but healthy. Bernadette's blog <bernadettevella.blogspot.com> has tracked her progress since her first diagnosis and through the ups and downs of treatment and recovery.

BERNADETTE VELLA: I got the cancer diagnosis the Wednesday before Easter and, the day before, I had just got the results of a CVS test [chorionic villus sampling, a common prenatal test]. They had told me that my little baby was a girl and had no chromosomal disorders. I had gone to my mum's group that day and we did an Easter egg hunt with our two-year-olds. I got home and felt very unwell. I was supposed to make Tiernan an Easter hat for a parade the next day but I felt too unwell to move off the couch. Eventually I decided to go to the hospital. At the hospital they thought I had a pulmonary oedema and they told me I had to have a CT scan or else I could be dead by morning. Despite being pregnant, I had the CT. While I was waiting for the results I really wasn't nervous, as I didn't truly believe there was anything seriously wrong with me. Eventually the doctor came back and told me I didn't have a pulmonary oedema. It was not even a feeling of relief — I really didn't think anything serious was wrong. Her next words shocked the life out of me. She said, 'You have cancer.'

For about 24 hours, life became surreal. It was like I could see and hear everything but it wasn't really me. Doctors were talking about cancer and treatments and terminations but none of it was sinking in. On the way from the Holy Spirit Hospital to the Mater (which was where the specialists I needed were), I swung by home (as you do at 12.30 at night when you have just been diagnosed with cancer) and picked up the stuff to make Tiernan's Easter hat. When I arrived at the Mater, I just focused on making the hat. There were a lot less tears than I would have expected — the information was just too much for my brain to cope with.

Once I woke up the next morning, slowly it started to dawn on me but even then I was quite calm. As the day wore on, the reality started to hit. For a while I suppose I thought they had it wrong. Once I had a biopsy and they had the results of that, I realised that it was not a mistake and it was really happening to me. The next stage was protection mode — here the doctors were, telling me that I could not keep the little girl who, only 24 hours before, I had been told was perfectly healthy. They were making me choose between her and me — the worst choice a mother could be faced with. I did not want to give her up. I have always been a person who wants it all, and this was no different. I wanted to survive the cancer and I wanted my daughter — there couldn't be a compromise.

A lot of friends thought I was in denial about my cancer. One even commented that I was the happiest cancer patient she had ever seen. I look back and wonder sometimes whether I was in denial or whether my determination to survive was just that strong that it beat out any negative feelings. I like to get my own way and get what I want. I usually succeed at anything I put my mind to. I suppose the cancer was no different — I was not going to let it beat me. I knew that as soon as it started to take over my thoughts and feelings, then it had won and I would lose. I don't like to lose — it is not something I do often. The cancer could control my body, and I had no choice about that, but it could not control my mind and spirit. I had a lot of anger (apparently that's a normal reaction to cancer) and I directed all of my anger and negative thoughts at beating the cancer. Physically I could only fight it as much as my weakened body would allow. But mentally it surely picked the wrong person to fight with. If I was going to die, then I was going to go down fighting.

There were definitely moments of feeling sad and sorry for myself, but they were truly few and far between. I always believed that if I felt down, then the cancer was getting into my emotions, and it was an unwelcome visitor there — it had invaded my body but I was not letting it invade my mind. I also felt like I was not just doing it for myself and my family, but I was doing it for all the other women out there who get diagnosed with cancer while they are pregnant. I knew that if I could survive and carry my daughter to as close to term as possible, and if she came out with no complications, then I could give others hope that a cancer diagnosis while pregnant doesn't mean the end of life for either the mother or the child.

After Arielle was born safe and healthy, I suppose the cancer took on a new seriousness for me as I realised it could actually kill me. At the age of 33, you don't expect to have to face your own mortality. Up until that point in life, I truly believed that, like so many of my relatives, I would be still going strong at 80 years old. My family has a long history of living long, healthy lives and I saw no reason why I would be any different. It really gets you thinking. The one thing I know is that I am not afraid of dying per se, but I am afraid of not living. It's a combination of not being able to live life to the fullest right now because of the cancer and not being able to experience all of the future, especially seeing my children grow up. That is what I am afraid of.

I sometimes wish I could see life through a two-year-old's eyes again. When Arielle was about three months old, I decided to have a photo shoot done of me with the children and my brain went into overdrive. I couldn't stop thinking about it perhaps being the only good family photo my kids would have of me. It got me very upset and in the end I was too upset to go. I was crying and Tiernan came up to me and said, 'Why are you crying and so upset, Mummy?' I thought for a minute about what I could tell him — I didn't want to lie and say that nothing was wrong but then I did not want to tell him the truth, either. In the end I came up with something that got the essence of what I was upset about without spelling out the details. I said, 'Remember last week how Mummy had a spider bite and it hurt Mummy?' He said yes, and looked at my leg to check out the bite. 'Well, Mummy is really scared that a spider might bite me again and make Mummy very sick and go to hospital and then I could not spend time with my beautiful little Tiernan and Arielle.' He thought about it for a few seconds and said, 'Don't worry, Mummy, I will protect you. If you see a spider, you tell me and I will stomp it. I will get my shoe and hit it and then it [will] be dead and [won't] bite you. I will protect you, Mummy. I will find all the spiders and kill them so they don't bite you. I will stomp them with my shoe — don't be upset, Mummy.' He then cuddled me as much as his little body would let him. It broke my heart and made me cry more, which I think confused him a little, so I told him I was crying because I just loved him so much and I was so lucky to have him to protect me. Then I thought, maybe he is protecting me. Although this journey would physically be so much easier without children, having them also makes my will to fight it so much stronger. On days when I feel I really can't do it, I think about the kids and know that even when I don't have the strength to keep going for me, I have to keep going for them.

When Arielle was a baby, she would wake me up in the middle of the night and I would be so tired I would just lie there for a few minutes and wish she would go back to sleep. Then I would realise that her hungry little tummy would wait for no one and I'd get up to feed her. I'd go in and feed her and she would look up at me with the most beautiful eyes and give me a smile that made everything else just melt away. At 5 a.m., when Tiernan announces that the sun is up and therefore it is time to get up, again I feel like I am just too tired to cope with it all. Then eventually I drag myself out of bed and, after watching Tiernan so full of life, I finally get on board. He is just bursting at the seams with the potential excitement of the day ahead. Or out of the blue he will come up and cuddle me and tell me he loves me and that I will get better one day (at which point I realise that he thinks about me being sick a lot more than I probably give him credit for). Even though sometimes I feel like I am too tired to fight this battle for me, I know that I have to for them.

A lot has happened since my diagnosis. I had a second tumour and my fight for survival became a pretty big battle. I got very close to losing my life and I truly, truly believe my determination to see my kids grow up and my positive attitude is what pulled me through. Only recently I spoke with some of the doctors, nurses and support workers involved in my case and found out that no one actually expected me to survive my second tumour and stem cell transplants. I truly didn't realise that I had fought such a huge battle and won. It was pretty weird to hear it, actually. I was told that the five-year survival rate is about 30 per cent for someone post-transplant. At first that was a little shocking and upsetting. Not only is there a good chance the cancer will come back, but I have an increased risk of other cancers and of organ failure due to the toxicity of the treatments I have had.

I currently have quite a few things wrong with me because of the treatment, but the main thing is that I am still alive. I am breathing and laughing and living life. Each day I get with my kids, family and friends is a blessing. Had I got sick 20 years ago, then I would not have survived more than a few weeks. I now even let myself daydream about seeing the kids start school. Tiernan told me the other day that he is not going to have children because he does not want his tummy cut open. I explained that one day he will fall in love with someone and marry them, and that person will be his wife and she will have the children for him. He is quite excited about this and talks about when he has his children all the time. A year ago I could not have had that conversation with Tiernan without being in tears. Now, though, I have the conversation and it does nothing but fill me with warm and fuzzy feelings. I plan on being there when he and Arielle marry the love of their lives and seeing them have children — my grandchildren. I have realised that cancer may one day take my life but in the meantime it cannot take away my dreams and hopes — they are mine to keep and cherish.

The time I get with my kids is a bonus, and seeing them renews my fight. This cancer is not going to beat me — I plan on being 80 and still kicking away. It is going to take more than cancer to take me down. When I decided to have kids, I took on a commitment to be there for them and to love and support them all the days of my life. I expected that life to be a long one and I am not changing that plan. I want them to grow up and know who their mummy is and the person that she is inside. They will never be able to truly know who I am unless I live to show them.

It's true that I see life very, very differently now. I rarely take things for granted and I take all opportunities I can. I try not to leave things for tomorrow because I am all too aware that life as I know it could come crashing down at any moment. I don't worry about the little things — I worry a lot more about feelings than I do about tangible things. I realise that family and friends and the love and relationships with them are worth so, so much more than money. I am currently surrounded by love and I'm the happiest I have ever been. Without the cancer, I probably wouldn't be this happy — which sounds strange, but it has opened my eyes and made me realise how incredibly lucky I am to be surrounded by so many wonderful people. I am in the unique position of nearly having lost everything I cared for but made it through — it made me realise what is important in life and what I want in life. Funnily enough, it was being told that my five-year survival rate was 30 per cent that was a huge factor in deciding to split from my husband — my time was too precious to waste on a loveless relationship. I was physically and emotionally tired and I didn't have the energy to support useless baggage. I have since met someone new and for the first time I'm finding out what it is like to be in love with and to be loved by a caring, supportive partner. If it weren't for the cancer I probably would have persisted with my marriage and continued to be unhappy forever. I've now reached a point in life where I'm truly happy and very satisfied with the life I have.

Strangely enough, I actually feel ready to die, with one exception: I need to be a mum to my kids for a lot longer — they are not ready to lose me yet, and my job with them is not finished. If it weren't for them, then I think I would have given up the fight long ago, but I have unfinished business with them. Maybe one day, when they are all grown up, the cancer will come back and I will not be able to fight it, but until that stage if it does come back, it is not winning, because God help anything that tries to come between me and my kids.

Dr Jane Turner

> *Being positive is something that is highly valued in our society and I don't think that is always a good thing. When it is something that comes from the person themselves, that is different, but when it is imposed externally — I have a real problem with that. I call it the tyranny of positive thinking.*

Psychiatrist Dr Jane Turner from the University of Queensland has a different 'take' on the question of positivity. In her work she specialises in the emotional impact of cancer, particularly advanced cancer, on patients and their families. You would think that positives might not come through her door too often, yet she describes encountering surprising honesty, intimacy and courage in the midst of dark situations. The flip side, she says, is that there is always a price to pay.

DR JANE TURNER: It is true that some positives can come out of cancer; however, that is at a cost. People will talk about the positive things as a way of avoiding going into the dark space to talk about what has been difficult for them. I think for anyone facing their own mortality at an existential level, it is almost impossible to take it on board.

The people I see are people who have been identified as having a problem; I'm a psychiatrist, so if they are doing flash, they are not going to come and see me. I'm referred people who are depressed or anxious, and the majority of my work is with people with a very poor prognosis, so I see a lot of people who die. I have a particular interest in families, so I see a lot of young people with young children. Consequently, the population I'm with is skewed towards the people who are least likely to say there is a positive spin. Having said that, the things I observe are that people will commonly reflect on priorities. They will say they have the capacity to let go of trivial things — how clean the house is, things like that. I see a lot of people who are depressed, and it's never just the cancer: these are people who may have experienced loss or abuse in childhood, or sometimes a series of major life events, or are very isolated for a variety of reasons. When you deal with the depression, you often have to look at these other issues. People say to me all the time, 'I look back and don't know why I put up with this for five or ten years.' Or, 'I think I've actually been depressed since I was a teenager' — so the cancer was the devastating precipitant that made them more depressed and forced them to get treatment, and it means they have had to look at other parts of their lives. But they can then feel that they have the capacity to cope with the cancer and perhaps other issues in their lives because their long-standing depression has been treated.

But these things come at a cost — and the cancer is the cost. It might also involve having to let go of relationships, it might involve having to make difficult choices. I recently had a patient who has been unable to work because of problems following chemo; there are positive things in her life but she is unable to work. She looks well, and the deficits are subtle, but they really impact on her ability to do her high-powered job. She did go back to work for a time, but it made her depression worse. We came to a mutual decision that this wasn't good, so she is off work till the end of the year. She related to me that she saw a friend for coffee and the friend asked about work and she said, 'I've got a certificate until the end of the year.' Her friend said jokingly, 'Oh, fabulous, can I go and see your doctor — I'll have a certificate too.' To which I replied, 'She is most welcome, but she has to pay the price' — she has to get cancer, she has to have a mastectomy, she has to have chemo. This has come at a cost.

From a medical point of view cancer is not as deadly as most people think. If you had to choose between breast cancer and severe heart disease I'd probably go the breast cancer because you are less likely to die from it. Even advanced cancer, where it has spread and cannot be cured — I've seen people survive ten, 15 years or more, depending on where the cancer has spread to. In many cases it is becoming more like a chronic illness, but cancer is such an emotive thing. You may remember years ago, the Cancer Council had a public awareness program: 'Cancer is a word, not a sentence.' I think in people's minds it equates to death. So I think cancer is a unique condition in that it makes people think about death. Cancer is cells that grow where they shouldn't, move where they shouldn't. At some level this conjures up an image of things decaying, rotting, things being damaged. If you have heart disease, your arteries are clogged, but I don't think it has the same connotations in terms of your body betraying you.

Often it has come out of the blue: I spoke with a person recently who had shoulder pain, then discovered she had lung cancer and it had spread to her bones and to her brain. The sense that you could have something going badly wrong in your body and not know is very traumatising. There are guilt factors about cancer as well, issues about smoking, diet — I think women who get cancer of the cervix sometimes feel ashamed and guilty, almost like they have a sexually transmitted disease. Women who have been sexually abused sometimes say that they feel dirty if they get one of these cancers — it is a complicated dynamic.

The whole 'positive' thing, from a psychiatrist's point of view, is a complicated issue. One of the things patients say to me during and after their treatment is it's a balance of trying to reconcile what's happened, deal with the fear it could come back but not stay locked in that state. Most people I see have at some level worried they would die, but they are almost universally pressured by their family and friends not to go there. Being positive is something that is highly valued in our society, and I don't think that is always a good thing. When it is something that comes from the person themselves, that is different, but when it is imposed externally — I have a real problem with that. I call it the tyranny of positive thinking. We interviewed 67 women who had been diagnosed with advanced breast cancer in the prior six months; a lot of them were young; there were a lot of very difficult stories. One woman said, 'When people say, "Be positive" or "You look fantastic", that is their way of avoiding confronting the fact that this has happened to me and they could be vulnerable too.' Doctors do it too; so often the patient who raises the concern they could die is immediately reassured — people don't want to go there.

I had a couple in my office; the woman had difficulty adjusting; she felt distanced from her partner. That is the typical dilemma for the woman with breast cancer: the husband who wants to fix it and gets upset because he can't. A woman has a mastectomy and he says, 'It doesn't matter' — she feels like choking him. What he is trying to say is that he can cope with it. Anyway, with this particular couple, she felt very angry that he had downplayed it. I looked at him and said, 'Did you ever think your wife could die?' She had a good prognosis, but he said, 'Oh, shit yeah.' She burst into tears and she said, 'That's the nicest thing you've ever said to me' — because he was acknowledging. For me that is a positive, that people can talk about their true feelings. You might think, what good can come from that? Sometimes you see people reconcile, and you see intimacy. I had a woman with advanced breast cancer; she had three children and she was really quite ill. She said, 'Look, I'm really angry with my mother, she's never been helpful.' We talked about it, and with some support she spoke to her mother; her mother said, 'I've wanted to help you but you've never let me.' So even with advanced cancer she got to the point where she could allow her mother to help and be connected. Now that is a big price to pay — the price was she was going to die — but something positive from that was she allowed her mother to be close to her.

There is a lot of magical thinking. When kids have a birthday, we give them a cake, put candles on it and say, 'Blow out the candles and make a wish.' You and I both know Santa Claus isn't real, the Easter bunny's not real, but we tell children these things as part of our culture. As adults, we don't have magical thinking generally, but when you are sick and depressed, you are more likely to regress to that level. I had a woman who said to me, 'I've decided I'm going to cut off contact with my mother because I get upset with her,' and I said, 'Why would you do that?' She said, 'I don't want it to affect my cancer.' People may resist making a will, because if they make a will it means they are going to die; people resist taking morphine for the pain because that means it doesn't need to be treated … I think people [with cancer] want to support other people because if they are confident, they will survive longer. That is a hugely common belief, but the evidence does not support the idea that a positive attitude will improve survival. The problem with the positive-thinking stuff is it puts a burden on them; it's not real life, and then if the cancer comes back, is it your fault? I heard one man say to his wife, 'Don't cry, you'll make the cancer spread' — people have quite distorted beliefs about this. I had a man who had a very serious cancer say to his kids, 'You've got to be well behaved otherwise Daddy can't get well.' What happens if he dies? Is it their fault?

Don't think everyone who gets cancer is a happy well-adjusted person — they are not; and family and friends don't always rally around. I had a family in this room with a woman in her 30s who had advanced ovarian cancer. I said to her father, 'This is difficult,' and he said, 'What's difficult?' I said, 'Your daughter has cancer,' and he said, 'It doesn't worry me.' I don't think I've ever heard another human being be so rude. His daughter said to me that her parents refused to acknowledge how serious her condition was: 'When I die they'll put on my tombstone, "Shit, that's a surprise."' Her death was very traumatic; there were family arguments and shouting — nothing positive about that. Even if things are really, really difficult, sometimes you can turn things around, but sometimes they get catastrophically worse. For health professionals that's the big challenge, accepting you can't fix things. On the other hand, I can remember a terminally ill woman in her 50s whose daughter was into drug abuse and promiscuity. They tried over many years to reconcile, but the woman reached the point where she said, 'I just can't do this, I've had enough.' I said to her, 'They say that if your toddler has a tantrum in the supermarket and you smack them, you have two people behaving badly. You mightn't like it but you are the grown-up, and this could be a burden she will carry for the rest of her life.' I guess I really pushed her; she was then able to say there was too much riding on this to let it go and they did reconcile. After the woman died, I got a lovely letter from her daughter to say that it made a big difference to her then — and it will for the rest of her life — that when her mother died they were on reasonable terms.

Cancer holds a mirror up to you and you are forced to say, 'Who am I? What matters to me?' I had a patient who was very obsessional and really struggled with treatment, with chemo. She said to me, 'I wish I wasn't that sort of person, I've found it difficult my whole life.' She'd been employed as a technologist in a lab, and I said to her, 'The fact you were obsessional meant you were organised, people got the right results.' That was the first time she was able to think about herself as a package, so for her, cancer made her more accepting of who she was.

Sometimes the kindness [of patients and of those around them] is at such an exquisite level. I had a patient who was dying and a family friend left a note that said, 'Until further notice, I will come to your house and feed and water and exercise your dog.' I thought that was the most thoughtful, kind and generous thing — just taking care of things, beautiful. I say to people that it's a gift; sometimes cancer can allow you to let people be kind to you. A lot of women with breast cancer have what I call 'confident woman syndrome': they are the sort of people who others look at and think everything is okay, everything is intact, so no one offers to help them. Cancer can sometimes allow those women to let people in; it is a good gift to their friends.

There's the person who struggles, has an affair, gets drunk, takes an overdose; the person who is angry and sues their doctor; and the person who is very mature and does things to help other people. But I think we can't always take things at face value: I've certainly seen people doing the 'mature' thing as a way of avoiding their own demons. By doing things for other people, it's a bit like, if you run fast enough you can't catch me. Busyness can be a way of avoiding inner emptiness and fear.

I see a lot of people who say, 'I can't be upset; I have to protect other people.' One of the ways I talk about that is to say, 'Don't begin to presume that they can't deal with this; how dare you make a decision on their behalf?' For parents with children, that is a big issue. That would be one of my big pieces of advice: be honest and let children see you are upset, because if you don't, you give them a message that they can't show their feelings either. One of the biggest gifts you can give your children is allowing them to experience sadness and other unpleasant feelings and know that they won't be crushed by them, they will survive.

There is nothing like cancer to cut through the nonsense. Once someone has been through that, you don't have to pussyfoot around because you can say it how it really is. And people draw stuff out of themselves that they didn't know they had. I see people with the most extraordinary courage. I ask patients, what would be the worst thing if they die? It's often about not being there for their children, but then you can help people see what legacy there could be. I had a patient who had young children and she died. I'd been seeing her and her husband and children; he came a couple of times after she died to talk about things, and he showed me a card. He didn't know his wife had written birthday cards to his children until they were 18, and it was their little boy's 13th birthday. The selflessness with which a woman can contemplate her death and for that boy to have something she had written for him, that is extraordinary. I encourage patients to keep scrapbooks; I say, 'What would you like to say to your daughter if she was getting married?' A lot of people never have that opportunity.

There are people who touch you, and maybe the positive isn't for them but for people around them. I've been doing this work for ten years and I learn from those people to continue to put my life into perspective.

Claire Harrop

Not a day goes by we don't think about [Angus] or we don't talk about him. [Our other son] Oliver talks about him all the time; in fact, he has become his imaginary friend, although he knows Angus is in heaven. We are very open with friends and with Oliver and speak very freely about Angus. I couldn't hide him away.

When Claire was pregnant with her son, Angus, she lost her mother to cervical cancer. In 2005, Angus died of a brain tumour at the age of three. Claire and her partner, Stuart, are planning to start a charity called Wings for Angus, and they have also raised $120,000 for two groups who helped their family through difficult times — the Children's Cancer Institute of Australia and Bear Cottage. Claire and Stuart have a second son, Oliver.

CLAIRE HARROP: I didn't think my mother was going to die. The nurses would say, 'You know, she is not here to stay.' When she went into palliative care I was still convinced she wasn't going to die. My mother was always a very strong person to me and I just thought, 'You are going to live through this.' She kept saying to me, 'I'm not going to be here for when your baby is born,' and I said, 'You *are* going to be here, because you are a strong person.' When I saw her getting sicker it struck me then, but it didn't really hit me until after Angus was born. I was quite numb in the first five or six months. When I started getting out and about and seeing other mothers and seeing them with their mothers, that's when I would break down — in the middle of shopping centres.

Angus was the kind of little boy that everyone fell in love with — I know that is a mother's response, but that is what he was like. Friendly, interested in everything, he had big blue eyes with very long eyelashes that would just take people in and they would fall in love with him. There was something about him that was unique — I kept saying he has been here before and I would always see my mother in him. Even when he was born I saw my mother's eyes. When Angus got older he would wake up from his bed and walk around a corner and I always saw my mother.

When Angus was three, he became unwell: he kept vomiting and complaining he had a sore head. I took him to the doctors, who told me to get his eyes tested. The next day I took him to a local hospital and they did a CAT scan and a blood test and couldn't find anything wrong with him. The next day I took him to Sydney Children's Hospital at Randwick and I told them I didn't want to go home until I found out what was wrong with him. The doctor I saw said she wasn't going to send me home until she found out what was wrong with him, so I was relieved. We spent the night at the children's hospital; the next day they did an MRI and found a tumour at the base of his head near his brain. They thought he had neurofibromatosis — NF2. The surgeon was going to take the tumour out and he was worried as it was very close to lots of nerve endings, so the operation might damage his hearing and facial muscles. All I could think was, 'Not his beautiful face!' They removed the tumour and he was in intensive care for three days. I knew he would pull through. We found out a few days later that the tumour was cancerous and he might have to go through chemo. Nine days later we took Angus home, which was a great joy for us all but especially [for] his brother, Oliver, who was so excited to see Angus — Oliver was 18 months old at the time.

We took Angus home on the Friday; on Saturday morning he was back in hospital complaining that his head was hurting, and he was vomiting again. Monday morning the hospital did another MRI and found the cancerous tumour was all down his spine and had spread through his brain. That afternoon we were told Angus would only have days to live. Two days later we went to Bear Cottage in Manly for Angus to die. We left Randwick Children's Hospital on the Wednesday and Angus died at Bear Cottage on Saturday.

Not a day goes by we don't think about him or we don't talk about him. Oliver talks about him all the time; in fact, he has become his imaginary friend, although he knows Angus is in heaven. We are very open with friends and with Oliver and speak very freely about Angus. I couldn't hide him away.

I think there are no positives out of cancer, but there are things that come out — you don't take life for granted. I know that is an old cliché but each day that I spend with my little boy, Oliver, I treasure every single moment.

One of the hardest things about losing a child and having another one still alive is the question, 'So is this your only child? I remember being at the pool where Oliver has swimming lessons — Angus went there, too. There was a man there with his daughter, wife and two grandchildren. The daughter was going to shower her daughter and left her baby with her father — grand-dad. He looked at me and said, 'I raised three children and now she thinks I can't look after her baby for ten minutes.' He asked me how many children I had and I said, with tears in my eyes, 'Two, and my eldest is in heaven.' He then said, 'I have three children and one is in heaven, too.' We both had tears in our eyes and told our stories to each other. I don't tell too many people my story but I think I chose the right person to tell my story to that day. We both had a cry and a laugh remembering the joy each child gave us.

Tali Foreman and Karen Johnston

> TALI: *The inner resources and inner strength that we see in our work is extraordinary. Sometimes [parents] are literally on the floor when they hear their child has cancer, asking, 'Is my child going to die?' Then they just slowly pick themselves up and go hour-to-hour, day-to-day or week-to-week, whatever it takes to get through.*

When an adult gets cancer, the struggle engulfs them, their family, their friends. When a child gets cancer, that flow-on effect is painfully magnified. Yet time and again their parents can draw hope and courage out of such a situation, and become stronger, kinder and softer as a result. Two members of the Long

Term Follow-up Clinic at Sydney Children's Hospital, social worker Tali Foreman and clinical nurse consultant Karen Johnston, describe the impacts of cancer on the families they see each day.

TALI: Even though it is the child [who is] diagnosed, no child comes to us without a family or a carer, so we talk about it being a family experience. When we greet new families at the door on day one, they often express surprise when they see how relaxed the other families are. The parents may be in the kitchen together or the kids [are] running around or it might be a bit chaotic. New families will say, 'Are these people not aware of what is going on with their child? Can they grasp the severity and enormity of it? How can they be so happy and normal in the face of such adversity?' Over days and weeks, sometimes months, families start to change their expectation of what is normal: hospital life is normal, a split family for a country family is normal — 60 per cent of families come from outside metropolitan Sydney. Usually their perception changes completely and they relax into it. They see that it is okay to have a bald child sitting on your lap but still laugh, or it's okay to leave your child in hospital but go out and go to the movies or have people over. We often see another shift when the treatment has finished. There are a lot of parents who go on autopilot when they receive the diagnosis and say, 'That is devastating. I am going to pick myself up and just do what needs to be done for the sake of my child.'

They don't want to talk about how they are coping emotionally because if they do, they will fall apart. It's only right when the treatment is over that they'll let themselves really fall apart and, for some, it can be quite a crisis. Once they've slowly built themselves back up, they can reflect on what they've been through.

We say to parents, 'You will cope and you will surprise yourself.' The inner resources and inner strength that we see in our work are extraordinary. Sometimes parents are literally on the floor when they hear their child has cancer, asking, 'Is my child going to die?' Then they just slowly pick themselves up and go hour-to-hour, day-to-day or week-to-week, whatever it takes to get through. When families and kids say, 'How am I going to cope?' or 'I'm not coping', I say, 'Look, coping is just showing up for treatment; if you are not coming for treatment, that's when we get concerned.'

Most parents who are going through it and do such a sterling job say, 'I'm just being a mother or father.' But eventually, when they do have the opportunity to reflect, they can say, 'I really did that, I can't believe I did it.' People learn things about themselves and the way they can cope with stressful situations that might help later on in life.

Kids as well as the parents surprise themselves with how well they can cope. We get kids from birth to 16 or 17, so it depends on the age group. Younger children tend to look just at the here and now. They can see a positive in being able to say, 'I'm going to school this week' or 'I'm getting to go on a special holiday through Starlight [Children's Foundation].' A lot of kids going into adulthood talk about having [developed] empathy for others.

Karen: People who have had hideous treatment sometimes see things [that are positive] now that they're on the other side of it. I am thinking of one patient in particular who came from a difficult background. Getting cancer led to her being linked into the services here and learning to see that there are wider opportunities in life, so she views her cancer experience as a positive one. She certainly saw it as negative at first, but now that she is through it and survived and is in her 30s, she looks at it as a positive influence on how she is as an adult and a mother to her own children.

Tali: The thing about cancer is it doesn't discriminate, so we see people from all walks of life. We see such a variety of socioeconomic status and ethnicity and religion and size of family and geographic distance from hospital. They are all going to get through it one way or another, but I don't think there is any way to predict who is going to let it absolutely consume them and who is not. It is certainly helpful if families are able to compartmentalise the cancer and say, 'This is one aspect of our very full and busy lives' but there are some people who just can't. That is not necessarily a bad thing; people do cope in very different ways, and you can't predict who is going to do better.

KAREN: Probably the most amazing thing I've ever seen, and it happened early in my career, was this woman whose child had been diagnosed with neuroblastoma, which is a really difficult disease to treat. She was from an affluent area of Sydney. He was an unexpected surprise later in her fertile life: she had this grown family and then this little baby she used to call her gift from God. He was diagnosed when he was about 14 months old. I was in the family interview when they gave her and her husband the news that he was very unwell and had a really hard road ahead of him. She burst into tears and went and sat by the cot where he was and stayed there. For three-and-a-half days, apart from going to the toilet she didn't move. She didn't shower, she didn't speak, she didn't cry, she just stayed there. We called psychiatrists in, we called all sorts of people in; her husband didn't know what to do, she didn't even look at the little boy. After three-and-a-half days she got up, had a shower, put her lipstick on — and bang, like that, all guns were blazing. She got through treatment beautifully and ended up being a major fundraiser. I asked her years later what happened, and she said, 'I don't know, I just shut down. [I thought] they can't possibly be telling me this. I didn't realise I'd been sitting there for three-and-a-half days — it felt like three hours.' She said that she just sat there and all of a sudden thought, 'I need to look after my baby' — and that was it.

TALI: There is an interesting shift that happens at that point where parents say, 'We are getting back to normal' and they realise that 'normal' is different to the normal they had before, and normal will never really be the same as it was before. They will always have that extra concern about their child who was sick, or memories of families whose children didn't survive. Occasionally people make radical changes; every now and then you get a wife who leaves her husband and says, 'He didn't really support me through this at all, so I'm cutting loose.' A lot of people will come to reassess some of their friendships external to the family; for some people that involves cutting people loose who they found really unhelpful at the time. For others it can be embracing new relationships — XYZ from down the road, who we never normally spoke to, was so helpful, brought around meals and babysat and transported kids. Or they might have new relationships they've formed in the hospital. Usually, changes happen in a gradual way.

KAREN: Sometimes I hear at clinic, say, five years down the track [after treatment has finished] that families re-established priorities. The dad might have been working seven till seven and not taking holidays and striving to pay off the mortgage; then they take a step back and think, 'Does it really matter if it takes ten more years? I am going to come home at five and coach soccer.' So there are some really positive changes in families. One mother who has five kids said that they never used to celebrate birthdays as a big deal; now they do make a big deal out of family birthdays because they appreciate another year. Embracing life, appreciating smaller things — I guess that is the shift.

TALI: Teenagers are such an interesting group. There are some really grow up quickly —

KAREN: — too quickly!

TALI: [The teenagers we work with] are often exposed to elements of life that teenagers shouldn't be exposed to: thinking of their own mortality, their own fertility, seeing other kids around them get sick, seeing their friends go on and do the HSC [Higher School Certificate] when they can't. There are some teenagers who really regress — I don't mean that in a negative way — they feel like they want to be closer to their parents and find the family unit the greatest comfort and just want to cocoon themselves in it. But teenagers are such a tricky group because they are at all different stages of emotional and spiritual development. If I am told, 'You are going to look after a 15-year-old boy,' I have no idea what I am going to find in that room. With body image and whatever going on, some of the girls in particular come out of it saying, 'You know what? I'm not going to take all that stuff so seriously.' Then other girls say, 'I've finished treatment, I'm going to my formal whether it kills me or not.' There was one girl whose prognosis was appalling, but she said, 'I'm getting to my formal.' She made a big deal out of it — hired a make-up artist, hired a limo, had the whole town out to see her as though she was a princess. That was really important to her. It was definitely a coping mechanism for her. She was insightful enough to say, 'I know this is a materialistic thing and I don't care; this is what I'm going to do.' And that is what got her through a couple of months of horrendous treatment — 'What shoes am I going to get? What gloves am I going to get? I'm going to have my hair done …' Goals are quite important, and sometimes they are small goals and sometimes huge; you just work with what that teenager wants to achieve.

KAREN: Some worry about things like losing their virginity and their ability to be intimate before they die, though they might not even be [in] palliative [care]. That is such a milestone, and it can be incredibly all-consuming.

TALI: Adolescence itself is meant to be the trial of who you are and how you fit in — and when you are in hospital 24 hours a day with your mum there, it is really hard to do that.

Celeste Powell

I think it has made my faith stronger and made me focus more. Before I was just a teenager; I was 12 when I was diagnosed, so [cancer] changed a lot of things. My priorities are elsewhere … My friends just have less appreciation for life, in a way, because they haven't had anything threaten that.

When you have cancer at the age of 12, your teen years can pass you by. Not long after starting high school, Celeste Powell was found to have Hodgkin's lymphoma. Now 17, it's been three years since her program of chemotherapy and radiotherapy ended. Although friends and family gave her strength, Celeste found there was a widening gap between her experiences and perspectives and those of her friends.

Celeste Powell: My first reaction was probably shock — it was all a bit surreal. It was hard because I lost a lot of my high school years. I knew I was different to my friends and going a different path; I had to grow up a lot faster than them. Some of them didn't know what to say; I guess I lost a few friends who I'd been close to. Some of them were supportive: I had a really supportive best friend. But being young, a lot of them didn't know how to react — they thought it was a death sentence, so it was a shock for them, too, I think.

I got a lot of strength from the people around me: family and friends. And I had a really good supportive church background and people I'd been going to church with my whole life. We were well supported with meals, and visits, and all of that.

There were definitely days when it was harder, but I had people around me. I always had a good prognosis — it didn't mean there wasn't a chance it could go wrong, but I was pretty assured all the way through by many people that things would work out and I'd be cured, so I relied on that a lot.

I think it has made my faith stronger and made me focus more. Before I was just a teenager; I was 12 when I was diagnosed, so [cancer] changed a lot of things. My priorities are elsewhere. I am still a teenager and still do teenager things, but definitely the way I think has changed significantly and is very different to a lot of other people. The way they see life and the things they are concerned with. I'm not in high school any more, I left at the end of 2006, so I have a lot of other older friends round me as well now. My friends just have less appreciation for life, in a way, because they haven't had anything threaten that.

Because I did radiotherapy in adult hospitals, there were workshops for women in their 40s and 50s to help them with losing their hair and getting wigs for them. I always thought it would have been easier if I was 40. The weirdness wouldn't have been there; I didn't know any teenagers who were losing their hair and I didn't look like a normal 13-year-old. I thought it would be easier if I had experienced life more, and lost my hair at an age where it was more 'acceptable', but in hindsight it was the best time for it to happen. I'm sort of glad it has shaped out the way it has. A lot of other changes were happening to me at that time anyway, so if I had gone through those changes and then had to change completely again [because of cancer] it would probably have been harder.

I was diagnosed at the end of Year 7, so I pretty much missed out on Year 8 and Year 9. Once I got back to school, I'd missed so much I don't think I could have caught up if I'd stayed. I don't think I would have left school [so early] if I hadn't had cancer. I needed a break this year, but I plan to go back to studying in the future. I want to do nursing. I have seen what nurses do and that is the area I want to explore. Or perhaps working with kids with cancer, or social work where I could maybe help kids going through the same thing.

The after-effects are hard; you can get through [treatment] initially but the after-effects are something people have to be prepared for. I'd want to prepare people for the bad days that come out of [cancer]. They are not all good, but it's not all bad. Cancer is not necessarily a death sentence despite what people may think.

Jason Garrick

It's not about pretending everything is fine; that's the biggest misconception about being positive in the cancer journey. Being positive is about being honest to yourself as well.

Angst and adolescence seem to go hand in hand. But for Jason Garrick, the usual dilemmas of girlfriends, exams and peer pressure paled into insignificance. When Jason had just turned 16, his father was diagnosed with metastatic melanoma. He died three years later. In those three years with his father, Jason painfully learned the value of honest tears, true friendship, and refusing to be defeated by circumstance.

JASON GARRICK: When your whole world starts to crumble you have that fight or flight reflex. Some people let it consume them, whereas others, including myself and my family, say, 'No, it is not going to beat us as well.' I got to know my father, not just as a father but as a friend, and I got to see some truly remarkable things about him as well as people around him. Because it wasn't just Dad [going through cancer], it was my whole family — Mum, my brother, Dad's parents, family friends. When they would crumble in front of us, when they would let their emotions go, we would encourage it. When you let go and stop holding it all in, it allows you to be positive. I think people underestimate [the value of] a good cry; you feel like crap, but the tears stop eventually.

It's not about pretending everything is fine; that's the biggest misconception about being positive in the cancer journey. Being positive is about being honest to yourself as well.

We knew early in the piece that this cancer was going to take Dad. We were told six months, maybe longer; Dad lasted three years and three months nearly to the day, with a cancer that should have taken him by mid-2003. I turned 16 the month before Dad was diagnosed. He took everyone aside one by one. He told Mum, told [my brother] Joel and then told me with Mum and Joel there, as I was the youngest and I think he thought I might have needed the most support. It was really great that he did it like that; it allowed all of us to be truthful, there was no hiding. When I was going into Grade 12, he had the major surgery to try to remove the cancer in the lymphatic system. Going through all that with the family together allowed us to be totally open with each other and Dad always said, 'If you feel like crap, cry.' I remember being told, 'The cancer is a lot worse than expected, he is going to have to have radiation, more surgery.' I remember just sitting there going quiet as he was telling us. As we were trying to process it, his parents walked into the room and he had to tell them. I walked out and bawled my eyes out on the sixth floor of Brisbane Mater Hospital. I let everything out, but it was time to start picking up the pieces. Cancer shatters everything you have, and if you don't let yourself feel how you need to feel, you can't be positive about it. We had an uphill battle, but being negative was going to make it harder.

When people say, 'Wow, how did you do it?' I joke and say I was lucky, I escaped a lot of that teenage angst. Because it just wasn't important. You are worried about your boyfriend not talking to you? I'm worried about whether my dad's going to get through surgery today. It really prioritised things for me. I got through Grade 12; I think Mum and Dad spent four months of school time in Brisbane. They were back and forth; they'd ring us, we'd ring them, our grandparents might come up and cook us tea — it was tough. Study was important and I still studied. Somehow I did really well: my results jumped up in some subjects, but not in the ones I didn't like. At times when I should have been motivated I wasn't; I was getting the whole picture together really. Dad was working in Brisbane up until he resigned just after his radiation. In the middle of radiation he was commuting to Rockhampton — 700 kilometres up, 700 kilometres back for a weekend. It taught me how to be self-sufficient in a sense. Of course there were teething problems, like Mum and Dad coming home and going ballistic because the kitchen wasn't clean, but at the same time it was a learning experience. I had to be older at home, to carry more of the load. It was tough but at the same time I got to have some awesome experiences and I really valued the time I had with Dad. A girl I was at school with lost her mother in a motorcycle accident, and I think, 'Wow, how lucky am I?'

After that 12-month block [of radiation] we had a bit of a reprieve. It just happened to be my high school graduation; we got through that, I went to schoolies, I behaved badly. He'd ring me up and say, 'How was your day?' and I'd say, 'I feel like crap,' and he'd say, 'I imagine you would; self-inflicted, of course.' That open relationship, being able to talk openly about the smallest of things, allowed us to talk openly about the biggest of things, and his cancer journey was so big and played such a huge role in my life.

In my first year out of school, Dad told me he had more tumours. I had just started work and he had to have more surgery. Then there was another lull right up until my brother's 21st and my 18th birthday. In that lull time we found out there were spots on his lungs; we started to get an idea that things were changing. We knew it but we didn't truly accept it. In that time we planned a party knowing this was probably our last big opportunity to do something like this. We had a big family lunch on 23 October, then headed on to my brother's 21st at one of the pubs in Rockhampton and had a really big celebration. In front of my family and closest friends, Dad said he was very proud of us; that means a lot to be told that.

Then another cancer tumour came up. It was the first time the cancer was outside that triangle of head, neck and shoulder; it was the first visible tumour. That was just before Christmas, and he said, 'No way am I spending Christmas in Brisbane this year,' so sure enough a few days before Christmas he flew back to Rockhampton. He was in pain, he was uncomfortable, but he was home. That meant a lot to him; that was a big emotional victory. The cancer fights your emotions so much — if you don't fight back, you will inevitably have a negative experience. He never spoke about it, but I can't imagine how disappointing it could be after you pour your guts out for a massive radiation stint and then find out a few months later it wasn't as successful as they thought and another tumour is there. I think Dad was very proud of himself that he kept on going — he never identified himself as a 'cancer victim' or a 'cancer sufferer'. He just had cancer.

I moved to Brisbane in February 2005 to study at the University of Queensland. Electing to stay at St Leo's College [a UQ residential college] was one of the best decisions I ever made. Dad was diagnosed as terminal in April 2005, just five weeks after I moved away from the family. 'Terminal' is a word you never want to hear during a cancer journey, but like many things through the experience, you have to pick yourself up and keep going. Dad told me over dinner after picking me up from college. Hearing that news ripped my heart out. I cried openly at college about it. Many people saw my grief and the impact it was having on me.

The final process of death lasted nine long months — with scares along the way. In that time we were able to talk with each other openly as a family about the issues affecting our lives. That experience is one I would never trade. Dad and I talked about death, relationships, love, life and what he wanted for me. We celebrated our final Christmas together in 2005 and he went into hospital for the final time on 2 January 2006. At 10.15 a.m. on 17 January he died. The moment he died, our family were all there. That moment will be with me forever. It was very bittersweet, the strongest moment in this journey — it was over. I was so happy that Dad was free from his pain and he was moving on. I was devastated he was gone. At that point I was very much at peace with cancer; it was part of our lives, my life, and it has positively shaped my life for the better.

I've had my pretty low days. Just recently with all the emotion, the build-up of stress from uni, the anxiety about milestones I was about to reach — I was on the floor bawling my eyes out for about an hour. I let it all out, I got up, had a shower. I cleaned my bathroom — that is something we don't have to do at college — and I cleaned my desk top. It was a small action, but you can start to clean yourself of the negative side of things; my way of kicking the emotional side in was physically cleaning. You find your little crutches to help you through things a lot quicker.

I used to cry at the drop of a hat; I was a 'wear your heart on your sleeve' type of person. I am a little more protected now, more cautious with my feelings and who I open myself up to. When I was about 16-and-a-half I realised I was feeling bad all the time because the friendship group I had wasn't supportive. I'd go to school and I'd just want to cry and I couldn't. That resulted in anxiety attacks, hyperventilating, the whole 'stopping breathing' thing. It was not a great experience, but a massive thing I've gotten out of cancer is that despite what happens you can get yourself back up, you can be positive and you can make what you've got work.

I started to learn how to cope with my anxiety and panic attacks; our guidance counsellor (or school chaplain), Joy, gave me all these great coping strategies: visualising things, putting them in a box, pushing it to the side. If you have to do an assignment, focus on the assignment; when you hand it in, come back to your room, open that box and sort through it then. So many integral things that I learned at such a young age: how can I say that's a negative thing from cancer? It is one of the most positive things I could ever have.

[One day at school] there was a bit of a food fight going on when I had this massive meltdown. It was a panic attack, I could feel it coming — hyperventilating, sweating, not being able to focus. I had a mild one in the morning and I repressed it a bit (learning experience: never do that again). I thought, 'I'll be fine'; I tried to talk to some of my friendship group about it and they just started talking about their boyfriends and how they weren't talking to them, and their girlfriends were being bitches.

I decided to go for a walk — breathe this thing out, just walk. When I had it under control enough, I went to the tuckshop and bought a bottle of Coke, but then on my way back I got hit in the back of my head with a mashed up bit of banana. I went ballistic. I turned around and said more swearwords than I'd ever said in my life at that point. Everyone in this massive lunch area just stopped and looked. I went nuts, basically; rage took over, I verbally abused everyone who had gotten to me. Just before this I had started to go out to functions, to parties and things, then all of a sudden I got hit with this banana and I went ballistic at all these people I'd started to have a few drinks with on the weekend. I just started walking away. One guy said, 'Look, he's going to go and have a cry now.' I said, 'You have no bloody idea; I think my dad is going to die right now. Just fuck off, you've got no idea, get bleeped' – I wasn't real creative in my adjectives describing people. Then as I walked off one person, Erin, followed me. She called out 'Jason, Jason'; I had a full bottle of Coke in my hand and decided to throw it against the wall. I split that bottle in half, so there was a bit of force behind it; the poor kid got covered in Coke but she still followed. She came up and said, 'Are you okay?' and I said, 'No, I'm not', and for the first time I truly admitted I wasn't okay.

I completely stopped talking to the friendship group I'd been with. I had been invited to go sit with a mate I'd met through tennis; a couple of others really came through for me: one of the girls was pregnant, so we were both having a bit of a crisis. They started to encourage me to be open, to be the person I am, and not hide it away. It changed my relationships very quickly: that was the first time I started surrounding myself with positive people, who are really the people you need. In the cancer experience, sometimes you have a friend who just does everything for you and then they are gone. It's not because you dislike them or they dislike you, it's more that they were there for you and then they walked away. And that's okay. Some of those relationships might have only lasted a few months but I truly do remember them.

You also have the choice to walk away from people who are being negative towards you, and that's the decision I made. At my 21st birthday, as I looked around the table I thought, 'Wow, these are exactly the type of people I want in my life.'

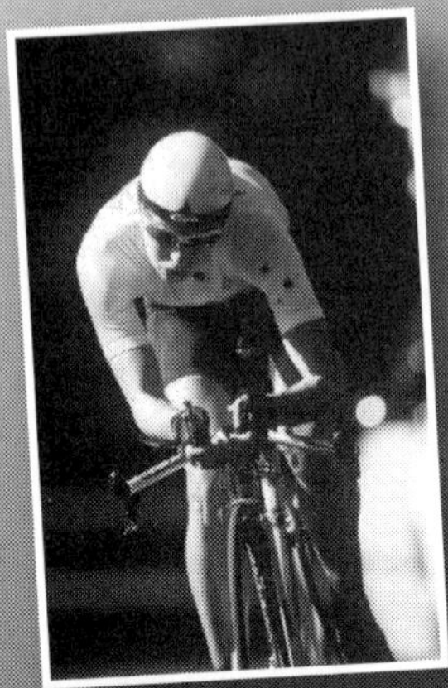
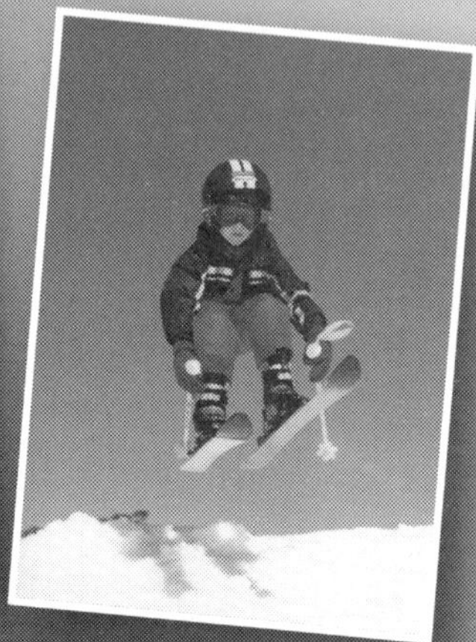
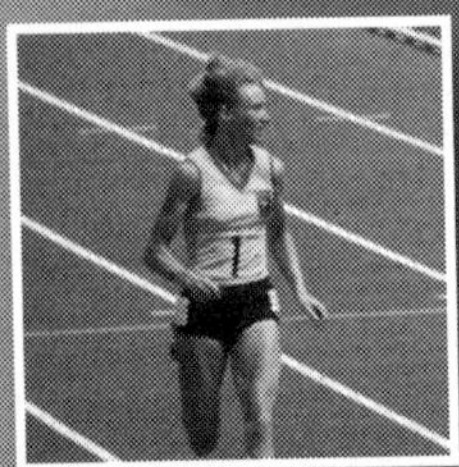
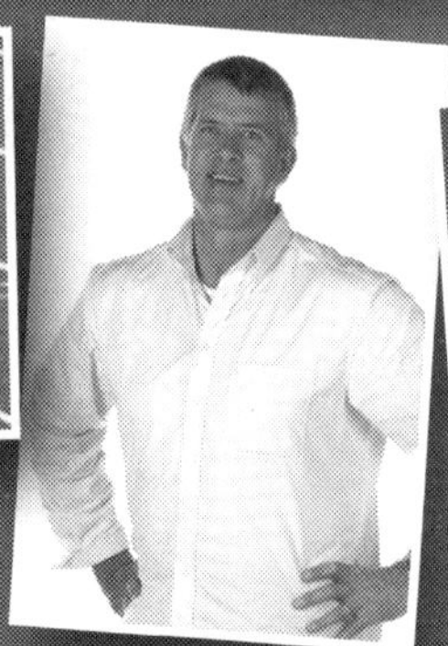
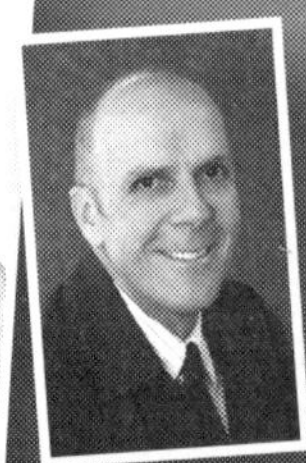
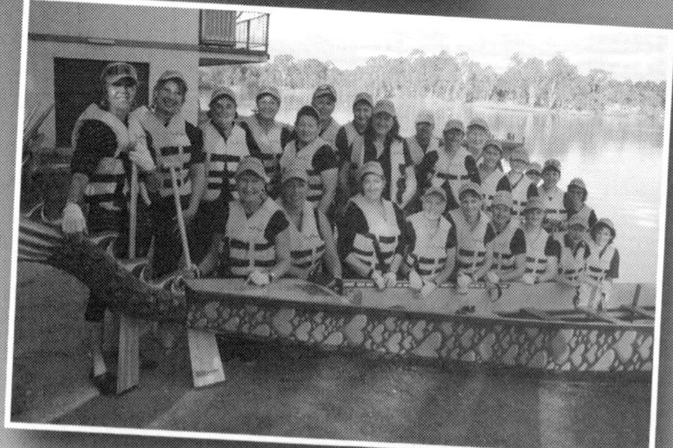

CHAPTER 2

The physical challenge

> As an athlete, when you least expect it, you may find yourself standing on the threshold of an accomplishment so monumental that it strikes fear into your soul. You must stand ready, at any moment, to face the unknown. You must be ready to walk boldly through the wall of uncertainty.
>
> **John Bingham, *The Courage to Start***

When you receive a cancer diagnosis, the physicality of it is immediate: biopsies, tests, scans, treatments, medication. People may speak of cancer cells as 'intruders', 'delinquents'; they may say, 'My body has betrayed me.'

For some people, the body issues go further and deeper still. Athletes, for instance, who are struck by cancer. Their bodies are the tools of their trade that they have honed and refined over years through purposeful, relentless training regimes. Athletes are used to being strong, in control of their bodies. Suddenly, that body betrays them, goes off message, entertains dangerous strangers in the form of cancerous cells.

When something like cancer hits, they become the weak ones — mentally as well as physically, when despair and fear set in.

Sporting excellence is not just about physical capability. Focus, motivation, attitude — they all figure in setting apart the gold medallists from the rest of us, and maybe that puts them in a better (or different) position to deal with a challenge like cancer. Track and field legend Raelene Boyle said, 'I keep trying to unlock what makes someone great and what makes someone [else] very talented but not great ... the ones who actually make it have this unbending focus and ability to bounce back day after day after day.'* Focus and resilience at that level are also ideal weapons for the chemo struggle, as cricketer Simon O'Donnell found.

Fear can be a great motivator, too, according to mountaineer Lincoln Hall. He used that fear to face off death on Mount Everest, surviving with his sense of humour intact but minus most of his fingertips. Fear of the unknown is what kept Raelene Boyle on her toes, both in her racing days and when confronting first breast cancer then ovarian cancer.

Once cancer is in their past, some people who were not previously athletes go on to seek out physical challenges. Maybe it's a celebration of life, or tweaking your nose at death. Paralympic skier Michael Milton is the fastest skier in the world — and that's after losing a leg to bone cancer. He

---

* Interview with Andrew Denton on *Enough Rope*, ABC1, 25 September 2006.

has also gone on to pursue speed on two wheels, winning a gold medal at the 2007 Australian Track Cycling Championships before being diagnosed with oesophageal cancer — which he is equally determined to defeat. Olympic cyclist Tracey Gaudry only took up cycling after completing a gruelling two years of chemotherapy, and she applied the same daunting determination to her chosen sport as she had to self-administering her chemo drugs.

Body image is also part of the cancer picture. Both women and men talk about the profound impact of losing their hair, or seeing their body wasting away under the effects of cancer and chemo. Performer Kylie Minogue, whose career and public profile are intimately interwoven with her appearance, said, 'When you are stripped of everything and you have to grow your eyelashes back, grow your hair back, it's just astonishing. It is hard to express what I have learnt from that, but a deep physiological and emotional shift has happened.'*

* *Herald Sun*, 9 October 2007.

Raelene Boyle

> *There's no doubt that there is a huge parallel between the experience of an athlete and the experience of being diagnosed with cancer ... The goal as an athlete is to win the event you are training for, whether it be an Olympic games or a Commonwealth games or a national championship. As a cancer patient, your goal is to survive the ordeal. In many ways I think cancer has helped me put my career as an athlete into perspective. I was just a runner; running is fun, running is something I drew great pleasure out of. But it was just a sport, whereas this game is dealing with your life.*

One of Australia's greatest runners, Raelene Boyle was the first track and field athlete to be selected to represent Australia at four Olympic Games. During her athletics career Raelene won three Olympic silver medals, seven Commonwealth gold medals and two Commonwealth silver medals. After retiring from competitive athletics, she turned her back on public life and studied horticulture, working as a gardener with a local council in Melbourne. Raelene was diagnosed with breast cancer in 1996, then with ovarian cancer four years later. Never one to turn down a challenge, she decided to fight cancer using all the resources she had gained as an Olympian, and to re-enter the public arena in order to help other people with their cancer journey.

RAELENE BOYLE: Before the experience of breast cancer, I had removed myself from the public eye. I'd taken on a much quieter life, in which I worked my job and came home and walked the dog. Cancer put me in a position where I could either be very quiet about it all or be out in the public eye and work to try to make the situation better for other women as they confront the issues attached to breast cancer diagnoses. From deciding to be very public about my experience, I've been exposed to meeting fantastic women — and men — who have lived the journey as well and have grown out of their experience, so that's definitely a positive. It has been a gift in the long run — not that I thought of it as a gift in the first instance, but breast cancer has given me the opportunity to use the profile I gained as an athlete to do good for a community that I love. Without my cancer that would never have happened; I just would have gone on my way, working in the field of horticulture and continuing to lead a very quiet life.

At the time I was diagnosed, the whole idea of finding a new direction was probably the most daunting part. I couldn't work in horticulture, which I loved, because I simply wasn't well enough while going through treatment, and I didn't want to expose myself to the hidden dangers of horticulture: the infections and the stabbing injuries from spines that you can get while working in the field. I was very concerned about my financial future and worried about how I was going to continue to have the nice lifestyle I had been enjoying. But then opportunities came along, and I've worked with some great people and organisations: AXA, National Australia Bank, BHP Billiton, MLC — the list goes on. So out of it came some great positives as well as, of course, the confronting negatives.

The positives weren't just for me; they were for other people, too. If you feel that you're doing something that is helping others, it's very rewarding for you as well. For me that comes from working with the Breast Cancer Network Australia as well as the Sporting Chance Cancer Foundation, Ovarian Cancer Research Foundation, OvCa [the National Ovarian Cancer Network] — there's quite a number of people who have been able to use my experience to help their organisations, but they have also provided me with situations where I've been able to draw positives from the people I've met.

Breast cancer has this amazing ability to link people — particularly women. We all share this common bond and we share each other's highs and lows. I see it as a unique situation, as is being an Olympian. Olympians can relate to how other Olympians feel, but the general public can't relate to being an Olympian because they've never been one. It's the same as having had cancer: unless you've been diagnosed with it, it's very hard to relate to that terrible time of diagnosis, treatment, and then survival — because survival is as difficult as all the rest of it. But I have experienced being an Olympian, and I have experienced being diagnosed with cancer. So when a person I meet has been diagnosed with cancer, I can say, 'I know how you feel, it's a shocking time.' For a person who hasn't been diagnosed with cancer to come up to you and say, 'I know how you feel' — in many ways you think, 'There's absolutely no way you can know how I feel, because you haven't lived this experience.' That's one of the big irks, for me.

People also say to you, 'Be positive.' I think people want you to be positive — and of course once you get to a certain stage, your confidence starts to grow again and you are positive. But at first, the fear and shock, looking in the faces of your family and seeing their fear as well — it's difficult to be positive when you're going through all of that. My immediate reaction to being told I had cancer was to think, 'I'm going to beat this', but a lot of that is in the lap of the gods. You go through the treatment that the doctors advise for you, stay on track, do all the things you need to do diet-wise, keep yourself stress-free — and try to keep yourself as positive as you can be. But I'm not sure that you actually elevate yourself to 'positive' status very quickly.

In those first days of diagnosis, you're looking your destiny in the eye. Being confronted with my mortality at 44 was certainly way before I thought it was going to be an issue. Some 12 years later I am still being a nuisance to everybody, but it is scary to be confronted with this word 'cancer', which to most of us symbolises the end of this life. I felt that I'd lost control of my destiny. You really do have no control — the doctors are totally in charge and you can't turn it around.

I have my days where I still suffer from fear and I sometimes wonder, 'Is this thing going to rear its ugly head again?' I call cancer the 'banshee sitting on my shoulder'. But I believe I'm a better person out of all of this, and I think probably the fact that it's in the back of my mind helps me get on with my life. There should be no sitting around.

It was the fear of the unknown that kept me on my toes, and it was exactly the same for me as an athlete. Fear was the driving force behind my success, because I feared losing a race, and that drove me to faster runs, to make sure that no one would beat me.

There's no doubt that there is a huge parallel between the experience of an athlete and the experience of being diagnosed with cancer. As an athlete you have a daily focus, which is your training program that you have to get through as well as the quality of the work you do. As a cancer sufferer, your daily focus is your treatment, getting through the day as stress-free as possible and moving on with your life. The other parallel is having a goal, which helps drive the focus. The goal as an athlete is to win the event you are training for, whether it be an Olympic games or a Commonwealth games or a national championship. As a cancer patient, your goal is to survive the ordeal. In many ways I think cancer has helped me put my career as an athlete into perspective. I was just a runner; running is fun, running is something I drew great pleasure out of. But it was just a sport, whereas this game is dealing with your life.

Simon O'Donnell

Initially the treatment takes away your control of your own body and its appearance. I remember disliking myself because of the physical state I ended up in ... I had a burning desire to become 'normal' again. It's about keeping a vision to come out the other end; cancer takes you to places physically and mentally you never want to go.

Multi-talented athlete Simon O'Donnell ended a promising Australian Rules football career to focus on cricket. In the lead-up to the 1987 cricket World Cup, Simon started to suffer from severe aches and pains and was diagnosed with non-Hodgkin's lymphoma. He brought many of the mental skills he had learned in the sporting arena to dealing with cancer. After 12 months of treatment, Simon regained his place on the Australian team; these days he is best known as a television sports host and personality.

SIMON O'DONNELL: Looking back, the whole period of diagnosis, treatment, all those things have been positive experiences, from the point of view of knowing what you are capable of — within reason — when you set your mind to it. It taught me a lot about the power of the mind. One thing you often hear from people is, 'Gee, I couldn't cope with that.' When you are set upon with whatever ailment it might be, in my case cancer, you actually *can* cope with it;

there is a mechanism that can cope, but you have to trigger the mechanism to *want* to cope. Often over the last 20 years I've spoken to people who have been touched by cancer either personally or through family members. They'll nod their head and understand what I am talking about — but others say, 'He's a weirdo; someone get a jacket on him and lock him up!' Those extraordinary experiences of the disease and where it takes you — it's only those in 'the club', as you might call it, who actually understand.

You don't forget it, either. The 'cancer club' works in two ways: one is a real sense of warmth for the people you talk to about cancer who have been on the journey; and then the people that aren't in the club, you actually don't want them to become members. You have a positive view looking back, but it wasn't always positive; it was done tough and you don't wish that on anyone, but you also know there are mechanisms to help them out.

To be honest this is the first time I've ever put anything into print, because over those 20 years I found it very difficult to do anything other than to sit down personally and talk to people about it. I found it very difficult to put it into words on a piece of paper because I never wanted to give false hope. I would prefer to be viewed as a person who gives genuine hope — for want of a better way to put it, I'm still here to tell the story. But I don't want people to have a false hope that, 'If we do what he did it will be okay', because cancer is the most personal thing you'll ever experience. *You* are the trigger to all the mechanisms that will help you. Your mum, dad, wife, kids — yes, they are support mechanisms, but the real mechanisms are within you and you have to find what triggers them to keep you going. I don't want anyone to reach for a book thinking, 'This is how you get better'; I think they've got to figure that out for themselves.

Those phrases 'think positive' and 'be positive' — it is such an easy thing for someone to say; it is different for someone else to go and do it. It's easy for a footy coach to tell his players to 'go in and get it' and 'be positive'; sometimes I'm sure the players think, 'Well, you go out and do it.' That is where respect comes in. That's with sport; cancer is a different thing again. I'll never forget the first time I was treated and my mum and dad were with me. When [the medical staff] put the butterfly clip in and turned the drip on, I'll never forget the sensation I had through my body; it was the loneliest experience I've ever had. I had lots of very good people around me, but in a way they couldn't help me: you are the one sitting there having to face that treatment. No one else can do that for you, so you have to gather strength from within to do it.

That was probably the lowest point for me, and that was good. I thought, 'I can't go lower than what I've just felt.' It was decision-making time that day: where do you go from here? Where you *may* go ain't much of a place, so all these people that mean so much to you are a wonderful motivation. They were part of the brighter side; the darker side wasn't a very pleasant place. It took that instant for me to face what was going to happen and what I'd have to do to get through it.

My personal way of doing that was to try to cut it down into small battles. I fought the hair thing initially; I said, 'I'm not going to lose my hair.' I did lose it. I remember sitting at home and a little piece of hair dropped in my dinner; the next morning my pillow was covered with it. So that was one battle, but I had to get on with the next battle and try to win it. They were continuous and constant, and some affected me more than others, but you had to think, 'I can do better with the next one.'

There is a Robbie Williams song ['Come Undone'] with probably the best line I've ever heard: it says, 'I'm not scared of dying, I just don't want to.' People said all those years ago, 'You could die.' I was petrified of dying, but that couldn't be my overriding emotion. If you continually think this is going to kill you, maybe eventually it will. If you let the [worst possible] result dictate what you have in your mind, it will be a tougher battle. It [worked better for me] *not* looking at the big picture; it was better keeping the little pieces of the puzzle and putting them together as it went along. I used to ask a million questions; I reckon the nurses would go, 'Oh, shit, it's Tuesday again, that O'Donnell bloke is coming in.' I'd be asking, 'What are you doing?' 'What is that?' 'Who makes it?' 'Who discovered it?' 'What are those butterfly clips?' 'When did that come in?' 'Was that easy to put in the vein?' The more I knew, the better I thought I could cope. 'How long have you been doing this for?' 'Have you ever missed a vein?' — and suddenly two hours of chemo was gone. They were coping mechanisms; I don't know where they came from, but something triggered them, and they seemed to work okay.

I was 24 when I was diagnosed; I was still learning about sport and how to handle situations. Although [cancer is] a different field, you can draw similarities — although the failure in this would be more grave than if you went out for a duck in cricket or didn't kick a goal in football. I think sport taught me to keep things in perspective, and to reason, 'It's not over till it's over; you are still in with a chance.' It helped me to [see parallels between fighting cancer and doing] something I was okay at, and while I was working within those boundaries I was comfortable in a way. You weren't thinking of the result, you were doing it bit by bit, knowing the result will look after itself — and that is a very sporting attitude.

There were lots of ironies. We went to India not long before I was diagnosed, and when I look back I knew [deep down] I was crook before we went. I wanted to go and be part of the team. If anyone's immune system is down or they have a cut on their finger, India is the place you will get pretty severe viral infections and tummy bugs. Fourteen of us travelled, 13 got crook and I was the one who didn't. In the end that was a strong motivation for me; I reckoned I had iron guts. Coming back I was physically in the best shape I could possibly be; my battle was going to begin when I got home, so it gave me confidence that I was physically strong — and I had to match that mentally. I thought I could come out the other end with no problems. I remember the oncologist said, 'We are going to hit you with everything; you are a young man, you are fit.' When someone says to you, 'I am going to make you feel absolutely shithouse and then make you feel better,' that is a very hard concept to come to grips with.

Initially the treatment takes away your control of your own body and its appearance. I remember disliking myself because of the physical state I ended up in — not through laziness or overeating. Whether that was me being vain I'm not too sure, but I had a burning desire to become 'normal' again. It's about keeping a vision to come out the other end; cancer takes you to places physically and mentally you never want to go. In the end you are proud of having gone there, but you wouldn't want others to have to go there.

And there are all the battles along the way; I remember Mondays going for blood tests and Tuesdays going for treatment and Wednesdays taking deep breaths and trying to keep breakfast down and get some normality, to have a couple of good days before I went back in the next Monday. It is a terrible place, but 20 years later I can say it's the most positive place I've ever been.

It wasn't long after I'd come out the other end of my treatment and got myself fit that I became captain of Victoria. I'll never forget that. Initially, I definitely had unrealistic expectations of others; I had very little tolerance of what you would call normal sporting injuries or aches or pains. I would look people in the eye and say, 'If you only met old Cyril or poor old Barbara, you wouldn't be worried about a headache!' I think I put the bar too high for the people I was meant to be leading. At the end of the day [I had to recognise that] it is just a game of sport; there is a winner and loser; you battle your bum off to win, but it's not a life-and-death situation.

When I retired [as a professional sportsman] I wasn't physically buggered, I was mentally buggered, and I think cancer had a lot to do with that. I put so much into [fighting cancer] in a short period of time. I always said to myself that even if physically you are gone, if you are strong enough mentally you can still get through. But the moment you feel yourself starting to weaken mentally, you are history. I felt that was the case for me as far as my career went. I had nothing more to give; I wanted to do other things, I wanted a fresh start.

Pauline Harbick

I often think we've achieved more in a group than we would have as individuals ... Our race is against breast cancer; it is not about getting in a boat and paddling fast and winning races, it is about being part of a team of people who have overcome an obstacle in their lives.

Pauline is part of Brave Hearts, a group of breast cancer survivors based in the border town of Albury Wodonga. Determined to be

more than just 'survivors', this group of women aged between 35 and 70 have built their own dragon boat. The boat was blessed in a traditional Chinese ceremony and launched in April 2006 — and it floats like a dream. In 2007 the Brave Hearts took part in the Abreast in Australia dragon boat regatta in Queensland, which attracted about 2000 breast cancer survivors from around the world. The Brave Hearts' message is this: 'Just let us know if you feel you are drowning and we'll swing on by in our 12-metre boat and lift you gently in. We'll keep you afloat. And when you're feeling stronger, we'll have a paddle waiting for you and we'll teach you to row.'

Pauline Harbick: We had a breast cancer support group which used to meet monthly; it was just a general support group, then somebody had the idea of an activity to give us something to do. Support groups can be difficult, because everyone who is going there has a problem, and the focus of the group is that problem. So our breast care nurse at the time had the idea we needed to do something with a more positive focus.

We did a calendar to start off with [for which members posed nude]; that was sold to the people in the local community and outside Albury Wodonga as well. It raised a lot of money and that was a positive focus for the group rather than a negative — that we all have cancer and how hard it is and how hard treatment is. Once that was completed we decided we would get into dragon boating. At the time Dragons Abreast Australia [which promotes breast cancer awareness, mainly through dragon boat racing] were doing a bit of publicity. It seemed like another positive thing we could do, so we ended up building our own boat and paddling it on our lake in Albury.

We didn't set out to build the boat. We had this money that we raised from the calendar and we thought we would buy a boat. We didn't know anything about boats or boating, it was just so far out of our field of experience. So we asked people from the local canoe club, and other people who knew about boats, about who would we ask and where would we get one and what would we do to get involved in boating in this town. One of the people we asked was a retired TAFE teacher, and for some reason he had this great idea — 'You could build a boat!'

You think of all the reasons you can't do it: we haven't got time or the skills, anything could go wrong … Frank was very keen and he believed in us, and that was really inspiring. He thought we could do it when there were a lot of people who thought we couldn't. It snowballed; this was never a project we initially set out to do in its current form — it came along in bits and pieces and now it's a big part of our lives.

If we had just bought a boat and paddled it, I think some people who got involved would have thought that it was physically too hard. I did a little sum yesterday: the average age of our group is 53 years old, our oldest person is 69. There are a lot of people who would have thought, 'It's sport and it involves upper-body exercise and I wouldn't be able to do that.' I might have been one of them, but having built the boat there is no way those girls weren't going to get in and paddle it. It was like giving birth to a child in a lot of ways: we created it, we built it and we are jolly well going to paddle it, and no one is going to tell us we can't do it — that we are not fit enough or too old or too whatever.

I think the community was quite amazed to start with. Everybody was saying, 'You are doing *what*?' and 'What is a dragon boat?' Now in Albury, when you say, 'We are involved in dragon boat racing,' they know what one looks like and how many people are in the team. It's been a real symbol of breast cancer in this town, and I think they now see that there is life after cancer. That is one of our aims — to show people that these days a cancer diagnosis doesn't mean your life stops. It does for a little while but it's not necessarily the end of your life.

When I was first diagnosed, I didn't know anyone else well who had had cancer and I thought, 'This is the worst thing that's ever happened to me.' And it probably is, but it is something a lot of people survive these days. Not everybody does, but you can live through it and come out the other end. It is pretty inspirational when you get to know survivors personally. It is a very helpful thing to be able to ring someone up and chat to them and say, 'Look, I'm not doing so well today' or 'I feel sick' or 'I'm not sure about this' or 'How do you know your cancer is not going to come back?'

The exercise part of dragon boat racing is great. But for me and other people, the support and belonging to a group is a very powerful thing. I often think we've achieved more in a group than we would have as individuals: if we weren't carried in that team spirit, there is no way everybody would have gone to TAFE to build a boat, and there is no way people would be turning up to paddle in the middle of winter. It is very cold down here — nine degrees in the daytime — and we are getting 25 or 30 people down to the lake to paddle. You really know something is there; it is more than the paddling, it is the group and the power of that group.

Our race is against breast cancer; it is not about getting in a boat and paddling fast and winning races, it is about being part of a team of people who have overcome an obstacle in their lives. If something happened and we could never paddle again, we'd probably be sad, but the group would continue to exist in some other form because it's almost like a family.

When I was ill, my friends or family would ring me up and try to understand and were very supportive, but I just got something from talking to other people who had been in this situation before. It is some sort of connection that I find hard to explain. It comes from some shared experience; there's a definite bond, and these girls have been like family to me.

We have lost some of the girls who were in the calendar. Belonging to a group of cancer survivors is a risk because not everybody might make it. But the group is still here and we remember them. Those people live on through the boat: all the names of the builders are painted in the boat, so we are [all] in that boat whether we are in there paddling or not.

We do get a flush of pride every time we look at our dragon boat. It's fabulous! It's really got a 'wow' factor because of the artwork on it. There were some things we couldn't do, like that painting on the side of the boat — the hearts and the pattern were done for us by a local company; they did that for free, which was wonderful. We've got quite a good local profile, and it is a positive one: we don't present ourselves as needy or victims or sick people, we try to present ourselves in a positive light. We are living life — we are out there, having a good time, having fun and we are making the best of every day, achieving something.

For our group, getting [to the 2007 Abreast in Australia regatta] was the achievement. It's not so much how fast you paddled or where you came, whether you won or lost. We had 28 survivors go, and we were training two or three times a week before we went, to learn to paddle to a standard where we were not going to look too silly and to get a degree of competency. The preparation and anticipation was probably as important as the attendance at the regatta. To get there and see they had flags and tents and people from all over the world, lots of colour, lots of excitement — it was a very busy event, too, so that was lots of fun. We all got to meet new people, people from other countries, and it was quite an amazing thing. When they paid their deposit to go, there were people in our team who thought they probably wouldn't [truly] be going — just in terms of being here and being well enough — but they made it. Everybody was so excited about it and we decided we would fit our lives around going to this meet. Even for me, it was a difficult commitment to make: I thought, 'How am I going to get away from this town for four days?' I have a child with a disability and I had to get someone to look after her, and I have a child who was doing the Higher School Certificate at the time, so I thought they were two good reasons not to go. Then I thought, 'No, the whole point of this thing is to do something for us and to work towards a goal and to do something as a team.'

It is never a good time: every day of the year you can probably think of an excuse why you can't go to Queensland. That is one of the changes that has happened to me since I've had cancer — it's the journey in life that's important. We are all very goal-focused, but it's actually how you get there that is more important. This is my life, it is happening now, and I need to live in it and do the things I want to do and enjoy it.

When you are diagnosed with cancer, that's the worst day of your life. Then it gets busy: you are seeing doctors, having scans, having chemo and surgery. All this treatment goes on for months and months — for me it was probably nine months — and then it stops and you think, 'Okay, what do I do now?' I really had a strong feeling that I just didn't fit back into the life I had before and that I was somehow changed. I was looking for something; there was a gap in my life, but I didn't know what it was. I was a bit lost and I think that's where this group came in. I really feel these ladies filled a hole in my life.

Nicholas & Lyndie Powell

If I didn't have cancer and the bone marrow transplant, I wouldn't be able to go in the skiing cup [for transplant recipients]. And if it wasn't for me going to hospital, there is no chance I would have met Nicole Kidman.

When he was 15 months old, Nicholas Powell was diagnosed with Stage 4 neuroblastoma, a form of children's cancer. A malignant tumour was wrapped around his organs; he was just days away from complete renal failure. Over the next year Nicholas had chemotherapy, radiotherapy, numerous operations — including one to remove the tumour — and, all up, 120 general anaesthetics as he endured test after test, culminating in a lifesaving bone marrow transplant. After seven long years with no recorded relapses since the transplant, Nicholas was given the all-clear and his family (mother Lyndie, father Mark and big brother Joel) could finally breathe easy. Now a young teenager with a sparkling sense of humour and energy to burn, Nicholas is an accomplished actor and a keen skier.

NICHOLAS: When I was in hospital and I was bored, Mum used to put on lots of Christmas videos. Then when I got out of hospital I went to the snow for the first time in my life, and I asked, 'Is it Christmas?' I kind of got it confused with the videos and I associated snow with Christmas. Ever since then I've loved the snow and I've just loved skiing. If someone gives me a choice between doing something in the sun and doing something down at the Snowy Mountains I'll pick the snow. I just like the feeling of skiing — I'm really confident at it. Last year I went down to Thredbo with Camp Quality. And every two or three years I represent Australia and Transplant Australia in a skiing cup in Europe. It's called the Nicholas Cup, but it's not named after me. [The Nicholas Cup is a skiing event for competitors aged five to 16 from around the world who have undergone a transplant.]

There are not many things I'm good at because I've got pins in my hips and [replacement] lenses in both eyes. I'm not a very strong swimmer so I can't go in races, and I can't play soccer or any sport like that — I can't play contact sports because I get worn out way too easily. I'm very short for my age. I'm in high school and I play handball with some Year 12s and they always hit the ball over my head, so it's kind of not fair sometimes. I don't really take notice of it, though. I'm really good at hide and seek!

LYNDIE: It's a bit of a problem when other people take him as six or eight ... We'll go to a restaurant and he'll say, 'If they dare bring me a kids menu and colouring pencils I'll scream!'

NICHOLAS: You'd be surprised how many times that happens. But I don't take it that seriously.

Along with the extensive treatment and operations Nicholas has had to endure, his illness and his time in hospital have brought some rare opportunities. He loves acting, and has been cast in several commercials because he can play the part of a young child while bringing to the role the maturity of his true age.

NICHOLAS: When I was in kindergarten, Mum saw an ad for actors in the *Bush Telegraph*, the weekly newspaper at my old school. There was a drama group held in the school hall every Friday. So I went and tried it out and I loved it, and I'm still doing drama now. I've done a couple of ads. I can do a part of someone that is a lot younger than I am. Instead of getting a younger kid to do it who wants to muck around all day and gets bored easily, I've got the maturity to do the part.

If I didn't have cancer and the bone marrow transplant, I wouldn't be able to go in the skiing cup. And if it wasn't for me going to hospital, there is no chance I would have met Nicole Kidman. Through the hospital, I was chosen to give a bouquet of flowers to Nicole at the opening of her movie *The Others*. I gave her the flowers and she put her hand out to me, so I just took it and she took me down the red carpet with her. Who else have I met? Michael Milton, he's my idol; he's got one leg, he lost [his other leg] to bone cancer and he's the fastest skier in the world. He's got the record at 213.65 kilometres/hour downhill. Straight down — scary!

The Nicholas Cup is in Finland in March so we are going over there this year. [Nicholas won his age-group race in the cup.] Hopefully I am going to win a couple of medals, but I'm not that good.

LYNDIE: He is up to the stage with his skiing where he needs to do some race training and discipline training — if I can get him a sponsor, because we are not in a position to do that. These cups come up every two or three years and we do them, but then we do nothing for the next two or three years to pay off the credit cards and get ready for the next one.

We make sure we do those trips; we don't buy things for the house, say. It is a priority to have those life experiences and do those things. I wouldn't say no to [Nicholas participating in] something because we couldn't afford it. I held a fundraiser to help get the team to Finland, and I'm going as team manager this time. We wouldn't be able to do it without sponsors or fundraisers.

I feel that Nicholas is meant to be here. He's a wonderful child, always happy. Through everything, he's always had a determination, and it makes it so much easier for Mark and me. When people would say, 'How are you doing?' it would be entirely dependent upon what was happening to Nicholas. If he was having a really bad time in the hospital with chemo, it wasn't so good, but if he was okay and having a good day — well, you'd make it as normal as possible. And we've met a lot of wonderful people; I think if he didn't have cancer, we would never have done the ski cup, the travelling and skiing.

Nicholas probably would have always skied, because we are skiers, but his ability level would not have been so high. But because he is in a different category, he can go in disabled and transplant events; it gives him opportunities.

Nicholas was invited to the launch of the Singapore Airlines airbus, and he and his dad went out. We are his entourage; we get to take him to these places. It's not a bad job to have, except I'm only known as 'Nicholas's mum'!

Although Nicholas has been given the all-clear from the neuroblastoma, he can't yet say goodbye to hospital. There are ongoing concerns with his renal function, and he has developed some benign tumours that require careful monitoring.

NICHOLAS: As far as the neuroblastoma goes, I've got another little one that is not doing much. They've tried to take all of it out but it is in a tender area. Luckily it's not growing or anything. And I've got an osteochondroma [benign bone tumour] — like a retarded bone. It moves — it was on my back and one day I noticed it was just kind of shrinking away, and the doctors hadn't heard of that happening. Then one day my knee started hurting, and I went and got my knee X-rayed and it is an osteochondroma. I've called him Bob.

LYNDIE: He still has big renal issues; he has only one partially functioning kidney and no urethras, he has an illeal conduit [a small 'pouch' created from a piece of bowel] which joins the kidney to the bladder. His renal function is dropping so we have to watch that carefully. If that starts to go in a hurry we are looking at a kidney transplant — which will be mine. So everything is great when it's great, but as soon as he says he has a stomachache or a pain here or there, you immediately revert to the medical practitioner. You can't afford to take anything lightly; you are on standby, it is always in the background.

John Stubbs

I am by nature very competitive, especially on the sporting field, and I carried that competitiveness into winning this cancer battle and not losing.

In 2001 John Stubbs had a bone marrow transplant to treat Chronic Myeloid Leukaemia (CML). A high-level all-round sportsman, he brought his innate competitiveness to dealing with cancer; for him it was a matter of winning and not losing. Since his transplant John has become a vocal advocate for cancer patients at State and Federal levels. He is the Executive Officer of Cancer Voices Australia and works as a consultant to the Leukaemia Foundation and the Bone Marrow Transplant Network NSW. John is also a member of the ANZ Clinical Trials Advisory Board; the ALLG Clinical Trials Data Monitoring Committee; the Therapeutic Goods Committee; the

Cancer Institute NSW board; plus other Federal and State government working parties relating to cancer and cancer services throughout Australia.

JOHN STUBBS: I was diagnosed with CML in December 1999. My prognosis was three to five years — a bit like a jail sentence. I suppose I looked immediately for the magic bullets: I sought changes that might assist to prolong my life. My partner, Julie, and I were in it together. We worked as one and looked at diet and meditation, because I think you need to be in a different place. Meditation did it for me.

Fighting leukaemia means finding someone with a blood match or a bone marrow match — that was the only course of treatment to cure me. In September 2000 I got the great news that somewhere in America there was a woman who was a perfect match. I was fit — in my youth I'd played professional Australian Rules, I'd swum competitively, I'd played tennis, never smoked, never been overweight, had a good heart–lung capacity — that certainly stood me in good favour. But I was on the cusp of being knocked back due to my age [52].

I had a bone marrow transplant on 1 March 2001 and I was in remission by May 2001. I was in hospital for 17 days, which at that time was a record [marrow transplant patients are often hospitalised for several months], and I was off all drugs inside nine months — again it was a record. I do understand my record has now been beaten; I will find out who it is and duly have words with them …

The interesting thing about a bone marrow transplant is that it is not like a kidney or a lung or a liver transplant where you will be on anti-rejection drugs for the rest of your life. My donor's marrow has kicked in and it's forging through my body and it's making new blood for me. It is definitely new blood because I now have my donor's blood group, and because it was a woman I am XX chromosome. It is an interesting phenomenon; things like that are good dinner party stories. During my course of treatment I tried to remain as fit as I could; I started taking supplements — selenium and fish oil and vitamin B and C — and fresh vegetable juices every morning. My clinician knew all about this and encouraged me.

[At the time] we had our own café and a catering company. Julie had been a corporate PR person and I worked for a large law firm, then in 1996 we did the big C change — café change — and never worked so hard in our lives. I was lucky enough to be covered by insurance, so I took 12 months off and Julie maintained the business. Café work is relentless and physically tough. I would not have had the physical capability to continue at that pace.

I was determined I wasn't going to 'get sick'; I didn't have pyjamas or slippers or dressing gowns, anything like that connotes illness. I wore bright T-shirts and shirts and board shorts in hospital, I had a variety of different brightly coloured caps because of hair loss. I had photographs and bits of artwork that were important to me in my room. Not only did that help me, it also gave the nursing staff a perspective of who I was outside that room. I declared that I was not going to ring the bell for the nurses [if I could possibly avoid it], so if I did, they knew I was in trouble and the cavalry would come rushing in. To me the important element was maintaining control, but there were a lot of people who were going to help me get through it. It became a real team thing, but I was the project manager. That worked particularly well for me.

I've taken a lot of those ideas into the work that I am doing now. I try to apply the skills that I learned and to bring the good experiences to other people with cancer. I started work with the Leukaemia Foundation; they had a consumer advocacy group looking at clinical and treatment pathways and getting patients and their partners involved in the process. That sat well with me, so I joined in. Three or four years ago the decision was made to form a national cancer advisory group [now Cancer Voices Australia], so I came in as a committee member and helped with its establishment, then I became the executive officer about 18 months ago.

Once you've had chemo, you get what they call the chemo moments, or petit mal [a brief epileptic seizure]. So you do lose a bit of confidence; you have to rebuild that. I didn't like the way my body looked after the transplant or the way my eyes looked after chemo, and other things you notice about yourself. Other people may not notice, but it's your body image — and it's a lot more intense for women. Losing your hair, that is the real issue; it's okay for a guy, I've got a good head, I could probably go bald, and if I have a look at some of the old photos I think I look okay.

[Through all of this] I never really thought about death. Going through the treatment, I always felt confident that I — and whoever else I could garner along the way — would keep me from dying. I know that I've got an inner strength that I didn't think I had before. I've discovered that I've got a very, very high pain threshold. I would have treatments, bone marrow extractions, for which people get knocked out for three or four hours; to me it is a ten-minute process. You feel this screw going into the bone — but I think that is where meditation helps, you go a bit comatose. I've made myself a commitment that I'll never ever go into hospital again, and for six years that's worked, I just don't want to be in that space again.

We kept a picture diary and I do review those images from time to time: from where I was then to where I am now. It's been a real quantum leap and I've got to be pretty proud of that. I am by nature very competitive, especially on the sporting field, and I carried that competitiveness into winning this cancer battle and not losing.

Tracey Gaudry

It was cemented in me during the chemo that if you want to succeed, you have to set your mind to it and you have to have 100 per cent belief in the outcome. That was one of the biggest things that contributed to the great success I later had [as a cyclist], but again it was one of the reasons I may not have won a world championship or an Olympic Games. Sometimes I couldn't just 'let it flow'; sometimes you can have so much focus, you waste a lot of energy on the focus instead of the instinct.

As a world-class cyclist, Tracey Gaudry has a will of iron. It shows in her cycling: within two years of taking up the sport she'd become Victorian State Champion and had ridden at the world championships for Australia. She went on to compete in three Olympics, win four national championships and 36 national titles and rise to be ranked 3rd in the world in 1999. Her strong will shows through in other aspects of her life, too: at the age of 20, Tracey was diagnosed with Acute Lymphatic Leukaemia (ALL). Given a ten per cent chance of survival, she has defied the odds in every way and is now a mother of three children.

TRACEY GAUDRY: I went through two years of chemotherapy, and two years is an extremely long time for having ongoing chemotherapy in anyone's book. ALL is classified as a childhood leukaemia; I was 20, and in 1989 the prognosis for an adult contracting that sort of leukaemia was pretty bad — it was about a ten per cent survival rate. At the time, constant chemo was the only way the doctors could consider completely knocking it out. Two years of treatment did the job.

For the first month of induction therapy I was in isolation in hospital because they were bombarding me with everything under the sun. The chemo was so strong I had no neutrophils [white blood cells that fight bacterial infection]. After that month I was deemed to have gone into remission, then the next 23 months was what they called maintenance therapy — I could go home but I was still on some form of drug every day for two years. I remained in remission the whole time, so a lot of the time it felt like I was taking drugs for nothing — a lot like taking out an insurance policy. It was a constant mind game to focus on the end-game, which was to remain in remission and make sure the leukaemia didn't come back in the two years.

People sometimes implied, 'The chemotherapy can't have been that bad if you could live at home.' But the chemo was a two-month cycle. Over a 61-day period I had maybe six different drugs, and this daily program repeated itself every two months. What that meant was that after two or three cycles I got to know the effect of each of the drugs, so my mind started to influence how my body reacted. For example, there was one treatment called a lumbar puncture, which was an injection into your spinal cord to put the chemotherapy in your bone marrow and your brain. That would cause me to have severe migraines for up to two weeks, to the point where I had to lie flat on my back except to crawl to the loo. If I got up, the pain was so debilitating I'd throw up. I remember one day I was determined to go to uni; I threw up all the way there, managed to sit through ten minutes of a lecture and nearly passed out while driving home. Once you got to know what was coming up, the sense of dread almost made you sick before you even got to that drug.

There was another drug called Doxorubicin — the name alone brings it all back! I would go to the hospital and they'd give me seven doses to inject myself with at home. So every day for a week I had to inject this drug into my stomach. Within an hour of having that drug, I would literally be over the toilet bowl for eight hours straight, to the point where I couldn't stand. It was absolutely diabolically hideous. If you can imagine that every day for seven days, every two months ... mind you, I'm on other drugs before or after so it's not as if I have a holiday in between times, but the week before the Doxorubicin I'm nearly sick just thinking about it. Every time I had to inject, it was worse.

Anyone would say I've got a strong mind, but it took every ounce of my mental ability to make myself do that. I had an instance of just one little ounce of weakness in me. One day it got the better of me: I flushed the injection down the toilet because I could not bear it. I swear I nearly went down the bowl after it to try to get it back. And for the whole two years I had this thought: 'If I fall out of remission, it is all my fault.' It was one injection out of 100, one day of treatment out of 700, but I thought that if I fell out of remission it was that one day when I weakened which [would have] caused the cancer to come back. I was so distraught because I'd done it, but I was so weak I couldn't take that drug. Every single time after that, it didn't make it any easier to take it, but it was a pivotal time. It made me remind myself, 'You are in control, you still have some level of influence; you can choose to take the drugs or choose not to, but the minute you choose not to, you are hammering a nail in your own coffin.'

Having been a young adult when I was diagnosed, [the cancer] catapulted me out of childhood and teenagehood into adulthood. I was brought up in a single-parent family, the youngest of three siblings. We had a very basic childhood, and Mum was very responsible: every single dollar went for us. Life was hard for her, it wasn't luxurious, and so we were brought up to be responsible — work hard, get a job, toe the line, not rely on anybody. I've had a job since I was 14 or so; I paid board at home at the age of 15 to help Mum just a bit; I worked to get through school. That's simply how it was. Even at uni I was working 35 hours a week at two jobs as well as full-time study. I was still having fun, doing all the social things and mucking up and all the things I believe you have to do as a uni student, but it was still largely a responsible life. Then when the leukaemia came along I thought, 'I haven't really had as much fun in life as I should have allowed myself at this young age, but I've got two years of jail to get through now.'

It was like a jail sentence. Every day there is something hanging over you; you are not free to do as you please; however every day is one step towards freedom and regaining a life to pursue as you choose. The funny thing is I almost never doubted I was going to make it — except for that one instance of terror. There was no doubt in my mind that the drugs and the program were going to work; I had no doubts about the medical team. I sometimes worried about not worrying.

During the chemo, I didn't want to be seen as a patient. I never ever took pity on myself. This is a lot of the strength of my mum coming through in me: never let anyone have to be responsible for you, don't rely on people, even to the point of being wary about trusting people — because at the end of the day you have to look after yourself.

I lived with the family of my then boyfriend for the first six months of chemo, and that helped me get through. That was probably the most dependent I'd been on anyone in my life outside of my family. My boyfriend's parents had seven children of their own and they took me in as well. They had all their own kids but they still treated me like one of their own. If I ever felt guilty about any of it, it was this — because they never expected anything in return. That probably had the biggest emotional impact on me of anything in my life: how people can care for someone so unconditionally. I don't think they ever realised how much I appreciated it; they never got anything tangible in return, they didn't get paid, they didn't get lots of presents to say 'thank you'. They simply gave and gave to help me get through, and I still often think, 'How do I ever repay them for that?'

After six months I moved back home with Mum and my brother until the end of my chemo. That was another special part of the journey.

At the end of induction chemo I enrolled back at university, which was absurd — I was so full of drugs. I couldn't spell my name, couldn't remember where I lived, but I was determined to enrol. I finished two degrees and started lecturing during the two-year maintenance therapy phase. Then I got to the end of chemo and thought, 'I have grown up too much.' Instead of using it as an opportunity to take stock, smell the roses and give myself a chance to realise the beauty of life, I had grown up and become even more responsible than I was before.

About six months after I finished my treatment, at the age of 22, I was lecturing to 300 undergrads, had started a Masters degree and was doing all these 'unachievable' things despite the chemo. I had a friend who was very perceptive and he said, 'Why don't you come on this bike ride? You need to have some fun.' It was a touring ride through Queensland, so it fulfilled my goal of getting fit; it fulfilled my goal of getting away from the day-to-day self-imposed pressure of challenging work and study; it fulfilled my goal of having a bit of fun, because I like to be active. So I borrowed a bike and went for a bike ride for a week; that was probably the first time in my life I'd done something just for the sake of it, without any real goal in mind, without doing it because it was the responsible thing to do.

While it started off purely for the sake of it, that is what led to my Olympic career. It is ironic because the rest of my life had been purposeful; I'd never done anything that had no responsible purpose. It enabled me to say to myself, 'For once just do something because you want to, do something because it *feels* right, not because it *is* right.' That was the most enlightening thing that came out of it. If I hadn't had cancer, I may not have done that.

I passed out on the very first day because I pushed myself too hard — riding 140 kilometres in a day on no training, after having had two years on drugs — definitely not performance-enhancing drugs, mind you! By the end of that week I had decided I was going to be a cyclist. Most people thought it was just a whim, but one or two people took me seriously, including the friend who took me on the ride. Within a month I'd phoned the Victorian Institute of Cycling coach and said, 'I want to be a cyclist, will you coach me?' She said, 'No, of course not — go ride your bike for six months then come and tell me you want to be a cyclist.' And in the space of a year I won the Victorian championships.

That bike ride was the catalyst: I decided what I was going to do and it was fantastic to be able to say, 'I am going to do it because I am absolutely passionate about it.' I believe cancer was a catalyst, too, but it certainly didn't bring an ongoing shift in how I thought and how I behaved and how I treated opportunities. It gave me more of a sense that you cannot control every aspect of your life, you cannot control your mortality 100 per cent; fate does play some part in what happens to you, so trust your gut instinct a bit more and go by what feels right. All the structure and planning in the world won't produce the best outcome.

One of my strengths is that dogged determination to get through. That can also be my undoing; it is so strong and powerful that some people can't cope with that. Since then I've learned it can be applied positively but it can also be quite detrimental. Not everyone is geared the same way; I've had to learn several times just to back off. While people can respect I've got the best of intent it can sometimes be too strong. So I'm learning that it can be both a strength and an impairment.

It was cemented in me during the chemo that if you want to succeed, you have to set your mind to it and you have to have 100 per cent belief in the outcome. That was one of the biggest things that contributed to the great success I later had [as a cyclist], but again it was one of the reasons I may not have won a world championship or an Olympic Games. Sometimes I couldn't just 'let it flow'. Sometimes you can have so much focus, you waste a lot of energy on the focus instead of the instinct. When I let my instinct come to the fore — that's what got me on the bike in the first place — that's when I enjoyed my greatest successes.

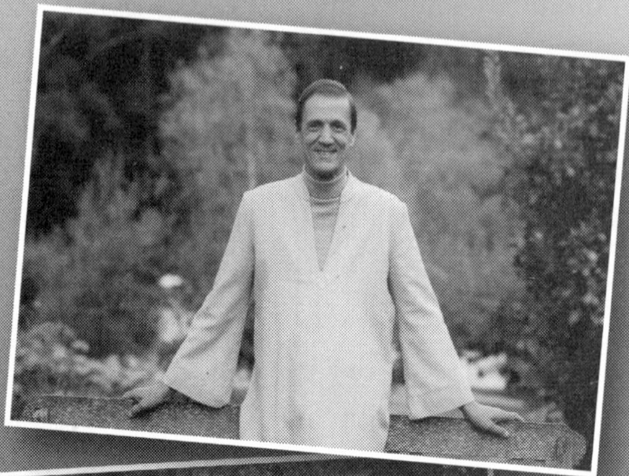

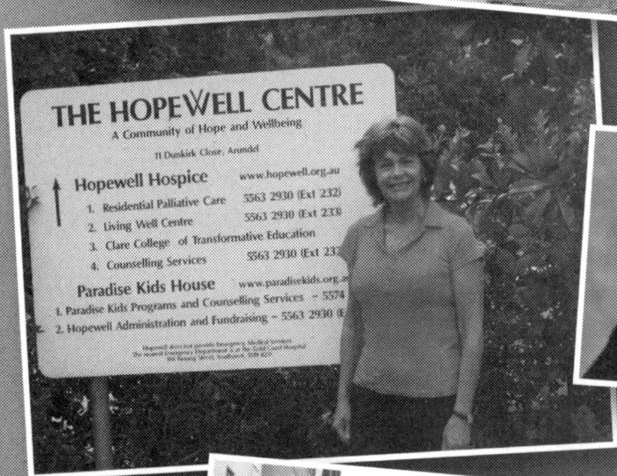
THE HOPEWELL CENTRE
A Community of Hope and Wellbeing
11 Dunkirk Close, Arundel
Hopewell Hospice
www.hopewell.org.au
1. Residential Palliative Care 5563 2930 (Ext 232)
2. Living Well Centre 5563 2930 (Ext 233)
3. Clare College of Transformative Education
4. Counselling Services 5563 2930 (Ext 23
Paradise Kids House
www.paradisekids.org.
1. Paradise Kids Programs and Counselling Services – 5574
2. Hopewell Administration and Fundraising – 5563 2930

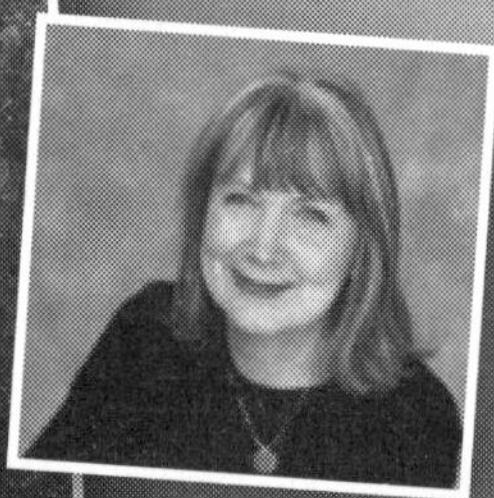

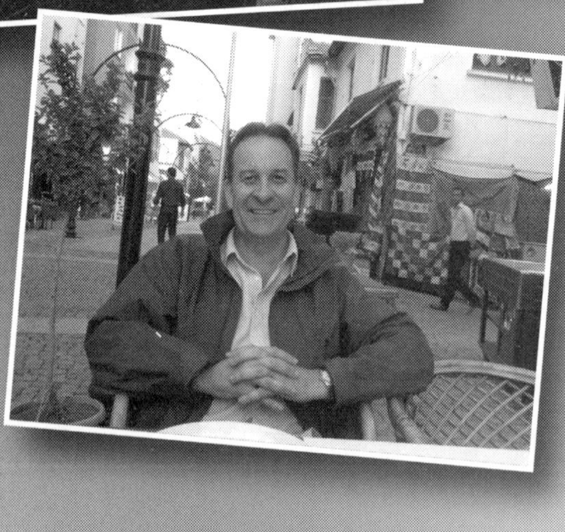

CHAPTER 3

The spiritual dimension

> In present-day Western culture ... the self is held sacred and death is considered an unspeakable insult. Yet the exact opposite is the reality. It is in the giving up of self that human beings can find the most ecstatic and lasting, solid, durable joy of life. And it is death that provides life with all its meaning. This 'secret' is the central wisdom of religion.
>
> **M. Scott Peck, *The Road Less Travelled***
> **(Arrow Books, London 1990)**

Much of what has been covered so far in this book is to do with how we go on as a cancer survivor, how we renew our vision of the world, how grief frames and transforms our relationships. But whether cancer threatens your life or that of someone you love, or whether you join the growing ranks of survivors, there can be very few people whose thoughts don't immediately turn to death as soon as the word 'cancer' is uttered that first time.

Until that happens, most of us make very sure to keep death at arm's length. Death is the uninvited guest at the party, the Grim Reaper leaning his scythe against the cocktail cabinet and waiting for a sign that one of us is ready to be escorted from the premises. But death also represents the ever-changing nature of things, the natural progression from birth and growth. Mind/body medicine pioneer Ian Gawler describes Western society as 'death denying', and points out that 'Buddhism starts with the premise that life is impermanent and could end any time ... It takes death into account right up front.' (See page 96.) Far from leading to a sombre outlook on life, Gawler suggests that paying attention to death in this way releases us to live life more vibrantly.

There are many spiritual practices that people use to achieve that more vibrant life, as this chapter shows. For hospice director Deirdre Hanna, it means delving into the work of the Christian mystics and going beyond understanding their work at a purely intellectual level. Actress Diana Davidson's 'golden key' is meditation. Donna Goudie sees the complementary therapies of visualisation and chi quong as her greatest resources. Tess Berthelson used prayer daily to help her deal with the treatment and found that her understanding of Christianity expanded, granting her a greater appreciation of life's inexplicables.

More than anything, cancer brings the wheels to a halt so that all we are left with are the most fundamental dilemmas: What does it all mean? What do we make of this? What does this make of us? Cancer can be the catalyst for all of life's most compelling questions. It can also slow down a busy life so that the shape of some of the answers may start to show dimly through the fog.

Dr Ian Gawler

> *Because cancer is a long-term illness for many people, it holds them in that state where they realise that death is a genuine possibility ... For the people who really work this out, what happens is that they start to live their life informed by death, rather than being in denial of death.*

One of Australia's best-known cancer survivors, Ian Gawler was diagnosed with bone cancer and had his right leg amputated in 1975. Later that year, inoperable secondaries were confirmed; he was given a prognosis of three to six months. Ian turned to diet, meditation and other self-help techniques and detailed his approach in the book *You Can Conquer Cancer*, which has become an international bestseller. A pioneer in the therapeutic use of mind/body medicine and meditation, Ian is the founder and therapeutic director of The Gawler Foundation. He now works intensively with cancer and MS, as well as conducting meditation retreats and wellness programs.

IAN GAWLER: The first diagnosis of cancer seems like a disaster in lots of ways. There is no doubt it qualifies to be called that. But very commonly the people I have helped over the years look back on the diagnosis of the illness and say it is the best thing that ever happened to them.

You may well think, 'How can that be?' In my view it is quite simple. It relates to the position death has in our society. We all know that we are going to die sometime, but there are really two ways you can live: one is in denial of that fact and the other is in full acknowledgment of it.

Our society is a death-denying culture. When you think you have an open cheque on life, it is easy to put things on hold, or compromise, or say, 'I'll do that later' or 'I'll get to that when I have got time.'

When people are diagnosed with cancer, it cuts through that delusion. It shocks people into thinking, 'If it turns out that I do not live as long as I thought I would, what do I want to do today?' People with heart attacks often think that, too, confronted with death. But if they recover, they tend to go back into that delusion that they will be all right.

Because cancer is a long-term illness for many people, it holds them in that state where they realise that death is a genuine possibility. Cancer is a much stronger 'gift', in that perverse sense of the word, because it actually holds you in the knowledge that you could die. For the people who really work this out, what happens is that they start to live their life informed by death, rather than being in denial of death.

Buddhism starts with the premise that life is impermanent and could end any time. Its whole approach to life is informed by death and it takes death into account right up front — the idea that life is very precious but you do not know how long it is going to last. So if you take that view — whether you are doing it from a spiritual perspective, through Buddhism or any other tradition that gets you to that realisation, or through having to confront death through something like cancer — it can bring much more vibrancy to your life.

Confronting death actually brings people alive, as they recognise the preciousness of each day, the preciousness of each relationship. For some people it is like an awakening.

In our group work, we often do exercises where we ask people this exact question. We say, 'If you only had three months to live, what would be the ten most important things that you would do?' When people write out a list like that, it is amazing how many things on that list they are not attending to. This is the list that reveals why getting diagnosed with cancer is helpful, and doing this exercise is how you can get the benefit of a life-threatening illness without getting sick.

If people are confronted with death and they do not have a good construct to help integrate it and get through it, that can be very difficult. I do not think that we are well supported in society generally to include death in day-to-day life. Society is much more geared up to protect us from death with all sorts of things, like the preoccupation with entertainment and being busy.

There is also an aversion to the painful job of working out how you place death in your life. How do you live knowing everybody you are related to, or in a relationship with, will die sometime? And how do you engage with people in an open and intimate way, without holding back, when you know they are going to die? We will all die one day; but we do not know when. You see a lot of parents who consider this reality with their children for a moment and just freak out and say, 'I would rather not think about it.' It is a very logical response; the problem is that if something does happen, most people are really unprepared for it.

There is this notion that to be positive you have to be 'up' all the time, and that to talk about death is being negative. It is actually more positive to be authentic to your emotions and to face the real threat that something like cancer can pose. It is more useful for most people to say, 'If I was to die and have a painful experience, that would be really difficult.' There is nothing wrong with acknowledging that. In fact, in doing so it can begin a process that can free you from some of the fear and anxiety, then you can be more capable to do what it takes to survive or get well.

Just as an example, a lot of people would feel that stress at work is a part of what upset their inner metabolism and had something to do with the timing of when the cancer appeared. I have little doubt that for some people, this is highly likely to be the truth. I would encourage such people, if it is possible, to take some time out from their work; to get a sense of balance and order back into their life, learn some new skills around stress management. What often happens is people then go back to the workplace and find that they can manage it in a different way.

Before I was diagnosed, I was a young veterinarian and a pretty serious athlete. I was working hard and playing hard. I used to have lots of fights with animals: the dogs would want to bite me, and the cats scratch me, or I would be having rodeos with the horses. There was a lot of confrontation with these animals going on. Vets often see animals at their worst, when they are sick or injured, and when they are unhappy, so on one level that is all understandable. However, after my cancer diagnosis I had a couple of years away from that work and was busy getting well, doing meditation and stuff, and then went back to work. It was amazing — in the two years that intervened, the whole animal population changed! It took me a couple of months to realise I had not had a fight with an animal. The dogs were coming in wagging their tails, and the cats were purring. It was extraordinary.

Cancer is a wonderful illness because it invites you to look at your whole life. It is a demanding illness. You cannot just treat it physically. You cannot just treat it emotionally. You cannot just treat it spiritually. Cancer invites you to attend to the whole lot. The good thing, in this sense, about cancer is that usually you get time to address these things; more so than some people do if they have, say, a burst aneurism or a heart attack.

There is no doubt that when I got sick I was one of those people putting my life on hold. As a young adult I made a fairly conscious decision to chase the material benefits of life and when I was nice and comfortable I would investigate what the meaning of life was. I had no doubt at some level the diagnosis was a commentary on that particular view as it applied in my life. I would not put that on anyone else, but in terms of finding meaning in my own circumstances there is no doubt that this was really helpful for me. That is not just hindsight speaking — even at the time it was as clear as day.

Before I became ill I had this existential dilemma going on in my life. I was working hard, I had my own veterinary practice. Each Friday I would go off to the bank with a nice pile of money and see my bank balance taking off. But each week, as I did this, there would be this little voice inside me saying, 'What have I done that's been meaningful in terms of my own spiritual development and personal progress?' The fact was, all of that was consciously on hold, and as a result, I was feeling a subtle anxiety. The illness cut right through that, as most of the things in the material world I was passionate about in those days suddenly became impossible.

Now if at that juncture I had dwelled on what I had lost through the diagnosis and the amputation, I could have had a really depressed, miserable life. I was fortunate to have a clear sense that going mad was possible and that I had the choice of how I responded to this. And for me, a key part of the solution was looking into how I could follow a spiritual path.

That focus lasted about six months after diagnosis, and

then I started slipping back into my old ways. I was just about to go back into veterinary work when, less than 12 months after the amputation, the cancer reoccurred. That added another level of intensity because it was clear from the medicine of the day that three to six months was a pretty definitive prognosis.

All the things that I could and did do for myself to get well had a spiritual undertone. Clearly meditation has that quality. Even seeing the sacred in something like food seemed both obvious and important. What this attitude meant for me was that the whole healing journey became filled with an awe-inspired joyfulness.

When there is something really difficult that has got the potential of being life threatening, so often it turns your life around. This comes back to that question we started off with: how do you live your life? Do you live it in denial of death or do you live it informed by death? For me, one of the realisations of the work I now do, and my own experiences, is that death is actually a friend, it is an ally in living well. If you take it into account, death keeps you vibrantly alive — thinking, 'I'm not sure how long I have got so I better make the most of it.'

Positive thinking to me is not some sort of vacuous process like wishful thinking. The mind is extraordinarily powerful. At the very least it is responsible for the choices we make: whether we eat well or not, what treatments we might agree to, how we conduct our relationships. Then the mind decides how we do these things — with commitment and enthusiasm or reluctance and reserve. Then, too, we can harness the power of the mind through techniques like meditation. Truly we can say that our mind shapes our life.

So positive thinking is accepting reality — and using our mind effectively. Being positive involves accepting the present moment, which includes the fact that life is both extraordinarily precious and disturbingly fragile; accepting things as they are; using our mind to do something useful; and living joyfully and fully.

Deirdre Hanna

Sometimes cancer can provide the opportunity for people to find meaning in their life. When people haven't had any challenges or big hurdles, they don't see the really precious moments in life, they have not stopped to smell the roses or be grateful for what they've got. Cancer can be a turning point or a wake-up call — though I think you have to be on a spiritual path to be able to see it like that.

Dealing with death has been part of Deirdre Hanna's life for many years. A former chaplain, in 1993 Deirdre founded Hopewell Hospice; three years later she started Paradise Kids, which helps children deal with illness, grief and loss. Even so, her own diagnosis with breast cancer in 1996 confronted her with mortality in a way that went far beyond her professional experience.

Deirdre Hanna: From working with people in cancer wards and hospices, I see that they either accept cancer as a part of their life that they have no control over or they think they have done something that caused it. That seems to be a New Age belief, that people have done something to create their cancer. Then there's a third group: people with a very high level of spiritual belief who see it is not as a curse or a gift, but something they can find meaning and purpose in.

Sometimes cancer can provide the opportunity for people to find meaning in their life. When people haven't had any challenges or big hurdles, they don't see the really precious moments in life, they have not stopped to smell the roses or be grateful for what they've got. Cancer can be a turning point or a wake-up call — though I think you have to be on a spiritual path to be able to see it like that. A great religious writer, Alan Jones [Dean of Grace Cathedral] says that two things can start people on a spiritual path — either a vision of great beauty or some great sorrow or pain, and I think cancer is sorrowful and painful. Physically it can be painful, especially if you go through chemo options and medical options. It is emotionally painful because your mortality is brought right up into your face.

Although there is that saying, 'Cancer is a word, not a sentence', I think it is still pretty scary. Death was my first thought. I realised I was one step removed from facing my own mortality. I've worked in the area of palliative care and hospice care for 20 years and it's always been other people's death that I've been concerned with, helping them deal with their death experience.

I had an obsession with death. I started talking about death from a very early age: in college when I was 17, I asked a group of students at the breakfast table whether they realised this was one meal closer to dying … It wasn't until I started working in hospice care that I realised this was my calling, to work with people who were dying. What I didn't realise at the time was this was also a calling to work with my own fear of dying. I had an awareness of death but it was at an intellectual level; at the soul level, the awareness was very deeply masked by fear.

I've done a lot of workshops in death and dying and spiritual care and nothing really prepared me for the statement that I had cancer. They did a core biopsy, then a fine needle biopsy, then the doctor called me in and told me the results. It was very aggressive and [I was told I had to have] a mastectomy almost immediately. I had a friend, Grace Gawler, with me and she said, 'Are there any other options?' and the surgeon said, 'No, not with this particular cancer.' They happened to have a breast cancer surgeon there — that was his day for visiting the Wesley Hospital — and he was wonderful, the most amazing person that I could have met at that time. Hearing that his wife had died of cancer, I asked, 'How long did she live?' and he said, 'Ten years,' and I said, 'That's a long time', thinking of myself of course, because that is where your mind is. Then I saw the look on his face and I said, 'Oh, but not long enough.' Then I realised the impact a cancer diagnosis has — not just on the person but on the whole family: my children, my grandchildren, the children still to come. So that brought up for me this huge sense of loss in my life. I really thought I empathised with people who were dying, but I did that as an external observer.

I know that I've helped a lot of people, but in this experience of my own, I felt so alone, so isolated from the world around me; people were out there carrying on with their everyday business, and here was I. A big cloud had suddenly come down on me; I felt immersed in this cloud; it took me. I teach about loss and death and dying and I knew enough to recognise it was the initial stages of grief, because a diagnosis brings great grief with it. So I went through the classic stages of denial and numbness and shock and disbelief. I didn't go into anger straight away, it was more sadness. I cried a lot; I cried and cried, and still this disbelief continued, probably for about six to eight weeks.

Inside me it was almost like the intellectual part was observing the part going through this range of emotions, but somehow they weren't integrating. I needed to go through the human experience of the loss and the pain and the suffering and the sadness and the fear until I could come out of it.

I had a great team of doctors. My oncologist recognised that because of the work I did my mind would go straight to death and dying. He said, 'You are going to need a lot longer than most of my patients to decide which way is best for you, because you only see people where chemotherapy has failed. Eighty-one per cent of my patients are cured, or at least I can get them to remission.'

At the time I thought I had created my own cancer through not nurturing myself, through not loving myself, being so busy helping other people that I spent no time helping myself. If you are constantly running on adrenaline, you lower your immune system. I would rush overseas, do workshops, and rush straight back here and build another building, dream another dream and keep on going.

I'm still rushing and still running because I love my work, but it's given me an insight into what it's like to be the person in the hospital bed as opposed to the professional. Empathy means to stand in someone else's shoes, so I must have been standing on someone else's feet but not in their shoes. Now I keep in my own shoes and I can relate at a deeper level; maybe not through words, maybe just through the experience that moves people to a different energy level.

I would love to have learned this lesson the easy way; I would have loved to have had the ability to read and study — to learn it the academic way. My intellectual side has been predominant all my life, but my emotional side was very underdeveloped. It is hard to say that, because as an expert you are supposed to know yourself — and I didn't, I didn't know this part of me. It was like coming back to being a child who just really wanted some help from God, but a little girl's understanding of God is very different to an adult understanding. What crisis normally does to spiritual development is throw it back a couple of levels. You see it particularly in children who are grieving, they go back to an earlier stage of development, and parents wonder why they've regressed: baby talk or wetting the bed or clinging, all sorts of dependency behaviour. A lot of people stop their spiritual development in childhood or adolescence, they don't move through to a high level of development, to the mystical level. I've read a lot of the mystics' work and I quote a lot of the mystics: Julian of Norwich, who says, 'All will be well'; the works of St Francis. I'd read them all but I hadn't integrated at my DNA level the mystical understanding of 'All will be well.' For me all wasn't well.

I'm not as scared now as I was in the early stage. I've come to an acceptance that I have had cancer and I am in remission. The thing about cancer is they don't say you are cured; if you have the flu you are cured, but they don't say that about cancer. They say, 'You are in remission', as if something is lurking there ready to spring out at any stage. But I don't dwell on it, I don't think, 'I've got cancer.' I've come to accept that this has been something in my life; it's been a wake-up call.

There is something in me which says, 'Lord deliver me from a sudden death.' A sudden death can precipitate people into shock and sometimes for the first time ever [have them] thinking about mortality and grief and loss. I think cancer is the beginning of a journey; that's what I've found in my life. In Lawrence LeShan's book, *Cancer as a Turning Point*, he talks about cancer as the opportunity for people, maybe for the first time ever, to sing their own song, dance their own dance, live their own life, beat their own drum. Some people might do that by spending all their money on a sea cruise or giving up a job they hate. You can take that risk because whether you live or die in the near future, cancer concentrates your journey fairly markedly.

Cancer is your own body changing its structure without you commanding it to do so. If I put a Band-Aid on something bleeding, there is a symptom there I can control. Some people will say by meditating they can feel the tumour shrinking, but for the first time I felt out of control. Cancer is like a juvenile delinquent of the cellular system. For me, I realised I can't control anything. I worry about my children living or dying but I can't control that. It has woken me up to the fact that I am a control freak: I'd love to control Queensland Health and make them give the hospice more money, or my son's driving, my children's eating habits and my grandchildren's eating habits; I'd love to be able to control George Bush and terrorists — but I can't, it is totally out of my hands.

I think ultimately all will be well. That is my ultimate positivity: that we are heading towards God, we are heading towards higher levels of consciousness. I believe we are heading towards goodness.

Tess Berthelson

When you have cancer, you are so drawn into the physicality of what is happening to you and the changes that has brought; I guess there is a hankering for something deeper. Interestingly, my spiritual life has achieved a broader dimension — as a Christian I now find myself less confined.

Tess was diagnosed with ovarian cancer in February 2006 and, after a recurrence in 2007, had additional treatment for tumours. She wrote to me, 'My responses to relationships and life experiences have a greater poignancy and intensity since having cancer. I find that minuscule details can be internalised in such a way that I feel quite elated, in a way I wouldn't have previously. I love this new richness in my emotional life.' Tess has been a teacher working in student welfare and has three daughters aged 18, 21 and 23.

TESS BERTHELSON: Initially for me, the spiritual changes involved meditation and quiet time for myself: I put aside several times a day where I would just be quiet and meditate or pray. I realised it was essential for me in that time of my life; I felt that was what enabled me to deal with the treatment and the things I was going through — to have time to allow that peace to flow. I had a sense sometimes of a greater being or other spiritual beings surrounding me;

that is a comfort and something which enables you to feel a part of yourself that is beyond the physical.

When you have cancer, you are so drawn into the physicality of what is happening to you and the changes that has brought; I guess there is a hankering for something deeper. Interestingly, my spiritual life has achieved a broader dimension — as a Christian I now find myself less confined. I've always been open to all forms of spirituality, pretty much. A literal interpretation of the Bible encourages the development of inward-looking groups of Christians that set themselves apart in an exclusive, even cultish sense. I can't relate to that, and since my illness I feel more of the collective spiritual consciousness, nothing in isolation. There is a bigger scope to the world and spirituality and life I can't even articulate. I feel even more strongly now that a lot of the movements going on in the world, both Christianity and other forms of fundamentalism, are just going the wrong way completely. We are leaving the whole idea of peace behind and pursuing something else, some sort of power thing. Or treating the Bible like an encyclopaedia, looking for something really definitive to hang everything on; I think there are 'inexplicables'.

If I hadn't had cancer, I don't think I would have taken the direction of seeking that personal peace, that quiet time and allowing the inwardness of spirituality as much. The whole emotional life becomes so much more intense — sometimes in relation to negative emotions, but in a way you feel you *can* deal with them or you've *got to* deal with them. Mainly it raises a whole lot of positive things — feelings of joy; you get in touch with your emotions in a really different way.

With my daughters, the difficult thing was telling them what was happening; I felt I was betraying them. Here I was meant to be protecting them and I was exposing them to the worst pain ever, in a way, but knowing that it was not my fault. I've written a lot to my daughters to try to explain to them. I've also written to them about the necessity of seeing that each moment is really important, that we've really got to live, that life is all we have, in a sense. That is for them to read now; I've also been writing them things that, if I was to die, they can read later and reflect on. It is a wonderful opportunity, in a way, to have that.

When I told my daughters the first time, I just blurted it all out. I've never been one to hold back on secrets. The second time round, I was really frightened to tell them. I thought, 'If only there was a way to just go on and not tell them; everything is wonderful and they are looking at me as their mum again.' When I wrote to them I said, 'I don't want you to see me as your dying mother, I want you to see me as your living mother and we are going to live lots of things together regardless of how long we have got.' I think after reading that and talking to me, they saw that. We've made sure we spend more one-on-one time as well as time all together. I'll arrange to meet Ingrid, who is my oldest, and we'll go to a movie. Sonja is my middle one; we had a couple of days away. I've always spent a lot of time with

Erica, the youngest, and we've continued to do that. I have always been that way — they would have a special day off with Mum, even in primary school and secondary school — but we have certainly done much more of it and enjoyed that time. The girls have their anxious moments; we talk a bit about that but not so much. Sometimes I ask myself if we are all denying it but I don't think we are; we don't need to go over and over it, we only go over the things that matter.

Once I'd been through cancer, I noticed you can savour the fragility of life; there is a different kind of joy that comes out of that. Just us sitting here now, or me sitting by that tree, or being on my own or with a friend or family, even watching TV — before I hated sitting around watching TV because I thought it wasn't constructive, but it is good just to be there and sit with my husband and grow more with him and our relationship. We've been married 30 years and we've certainly had our ups and downs — we had a few issues years ago, but we worked through that and everything is back on track. My husband is a wonderful companion and I realise how much he stands by me. The little things do become big things, but now you are able to see them in perspective and just enjoy the intensity of the love and caring that is around you.

I've certainly been at a point where all that was in my head was cancer. It was everywhere I looked: I could look at a wall and think, 'I won't see that again, I'll be dead tomorrow.' Emily Dickinson is one of my favourite poets and she wrote, 'Hope is the thing with feathers that perches in the soul.' I had to get that back, the flutter of joy that can always be there if you have hope. Things like that turned me around. I started writing a bit about cancer, how I hated the way people said they 'lost their battle' with cancer. That was always something that grated with me. I saw it as a dance. I'm dancing my way through life: sometimes I'm twirling fast, sometimes I'm collapsed on the side, other times I'm engaged with everybody, other times I'm just on my own, moving to music. That's how I want to be seen; I don't want you to talk about 'my battle'. Not very long ago I read Doris Brett's book [*Eating the Underworld*] and she said something about how she saw it as a dance and I thought, 'She heard me!'

There are many things that are still the same about me [as before my diagnosis] but a lot of things are more intense now. I've grown more in my understanding of my relationships and my commitment to social justice and peace in the world. And I'll continue with that as much as I can. I realised the value in relationship before, but now because of that poignancy, the intensity when you are with others in that moment, you see the importance in it all. My capacity just to sit and be is much better. Initially with the treatment, I was depressed and often agitated, but once I'd come through that I settled and was able to just enjoy.

I can appreciate more the place where I live; my husband gave me binoculars for my birthday, which is great because I love looking at birds and animals. I want to write; I've always been a bit of a poet, but I can't stop writing haikus. It just struck me the other day that, of course, a haiku is about capturing the moment, and then it connected with living in the moment. So in that way I've changed, too, because to be able to really intensely explore myself in a more serene way used not to be me. It was not me to sit and look at the TV; I'd say, 'I'd better go and do something.' I've always loved listening to music and now that has become really wonderful to me, I can't get enough of it. I have found that music has a whole different effect on me — it's hard to put into words.

My attitude to death has shifted only in the sense you feel a little more afraid of it. Leaving my daughters and leaving them with the pain. To see the pain in their eyes is really, really difficult to deal with. Everybody thinks, 'What if I was in a car accident, what would happen to my family?' but when you are faced with it, it's difficult to think of that and mull over it. As far as dying goes, I guess belonging has become more important to me, not just to people but to place — to [my home in] Hoddles Creek. I want to die there. Once I got sick and I was away from there, I realised that it was important to go to the place where my soul belongs.

Six months after this interview was completed, Tess Berthelson's husband Peter emailed me to say: *'It is with a very sad heart that I let you know that Tess finished her dance on 22 March 2008 … we have lost a part of us.'*

Donna Goudie

> *What I am shooting for is a miracle. I am very definite about that. I want spontaneous remission. There has never been a spontaneous remission with ovarian cancer, ever. That's fine, that just hardens my resolve … Whether it is meant to happen or not I have no idea, but I just believe it is possible.*

Donna considers that her one job in life is healing cancer. Her current medical status is 'incurable ovarian cancer', but she is aiming for nothing less than a miracle. The cancer was detected in 2006 after nine months of incorrect diagnoses, and in 2007 Donna embarked on a drug trial for women with advanced incurable ovarian cancer. She says, 'It's very early days for this drug, but the fact that it has appeared exactly when I needed it is not lost on me ... For the first time in years I feel "in tune" with life.'

DONNA GOUDIE: Cancer just turns your life on its head. From the time we are small kids, we live such limited lives: what our parents tell us, and what school does to us, and what everyone tells us life should be. Then you get cancer and suddenly for the first time you make your own decision on what life is. It is like a window opening: you think, 'I've been travelling along the whole time and it wasn't my life.' Cultural, social rules, all that stuff just falls away. You say,

'Wait a minute, before I die I want to live!' Nothing can fake the reality of knowing you are going to die. I think I was seven or eight when it hit me, burying a pet, that the rules said I was going to die at some point. I found that horrendous and scary but you put it out of your mind.

Even in hospital it didn't hit me; I thought, 'Thank God they've finally found what it is.' For nine months I'd been going to the doctor in agony and I kept getting told it was irritable bowel syndrome, so when they finally told me it was ovarian cancer, I was actually relieved. I couldn't have cared less what it was, I just wanted the pain to stop. But after a week or so the surgeon had to bring me back down to the ground; he told me it was really bad and I was going to die. The biggest thought I had was that I wanted to become more myself before I died. I was lazy, I thought I had heaps of time and just presumed I would have the average life span of 70 or 80 at least. I thought, 'Oh, shit, it's here knocking on the door and I didn't get enlightened.' It does put the pressure on — I would have taken so many more risks, I would have struck out much more, I would have been so true to myself.

That feeling has quite turned around now; that was a year ago, and a year is a long time. It's funny how a year can be long or short, but this year has been amazing. This is the gift of cancer, the way I see it: we know we are going to die, but we've got some time. Some people don't get as much time — I've had a year so far, I might get another six months. I want to counter this by saying that I believe and I am hanging out for that miracle, a spontaneous remission.

Now I stay open to anything people suggest to me and I have a look at things which I would never have done before. If I wind the clock back, one of my favourite sayings used to be, 'Damn tree-hugging hippy crystal-gazing' — I really made fun of all that stuff. I am looking around my healing room now and I have little crystals and everything, it's wonderful!

I'm more open-minded and I've got so much egg on my face … I am really analytical; I work in IT and I like things to be proven, and I didn't see any proof in that stuff, but now I know there is amazing proof. Quantum science brought validity to the alternative, or complementary, healing world. I don't know if I can articulate it all here, but every cell in your being is vibrating. Our vision is a result of vibration, our hearing is a result of vibration — all of our senses are, and our minds. There is a theory that cancer could occur where you've got suppressed memories and emotions in different cells in your body. You don't just store them in your brain, you store them all through your body, and if you can unlock some of those then the cancer will go away. Whether it takes cancer away or not, this journey work is phenomenal — the healing and emotions that come from it.

The motivation of having cancer has made me really approach [complementary therapies] in a studious way; I devote part of every day to learning. When you look at what homeopathy is, for instance, it works on a vibrational level; most people don't understand how it works but they give it a shot. I started taking homeopathic treatments for nausea and headaches. I've had three different lots of chemo now; they give you an intravenous drug that stops the nausea, but that drug gives you constipation and constipation itself is awful, so they give you another one to stop the constipation. This is what you find with conventional medicine all the time — they give you a drug to stop the side effects. It is just revolting and you feel poisoned. So I gave homeopathy a shot and it took me a while, but I was getting my oncologist to stop one drug after another after another. The last one to go was the nausea drug; I said, 'Can we do an experiment and try to use homeopathy for that?' It worked, so with my last lot of chemo I had no drugs whatsoever except the chemo itself.

I am not as disciplined as I would like to be, but at the moment I'm not doing chemo, I'm not on this trial — I'm not anywhere. My tummy is getting bigger every day, I've got pains and I'm having trouble going to the toilet. I've been through this cycle before and I know what it is: the tumours are growing inside me, and if you let your head go, that can be a bit freaky. But I know what my weapons are — visualisation and meditation and chi quong, and there are so many options and opportunities to give them a try.

What I am shooting for is a miracle. I am very definite about that. I want spontaneous remission. There has never been a spontaneous remission with ovarian cancer, ever. That's fine, that just hardens my resolve; everything I'm learning tells me anything is possible. Whether it is meant to happen or not I have no idea, but I just believe it is possible.

The most important thing is to have that belief; sometimes I get a bit out of touch with it and the fear grows, which is to be expected. I was having meditation yesterday and it suddenly bubbled up from within me — deep down there is a part of me that doesn't believe it is going to work. So then somehow in my meditation I dive into that part of me and I uncover that, layer upon layer, I get deeper and deeper. It takes you deep into your own worthiness.

I don't think we are brought up with the skill of introspection and it is not encouraged in our daily lives. We can go on completely deadened to what is going on inside us, when we really should dive in and have a look at what is going on inside. I want a huge amazing miracle and I've got to believe I'm worthy of it. It's like when you were a little girl and you wanted to be a movie star, but then you think, 'Everyone wants to be a movie star, what makes you think you are so special?' Hey, I want to find a cure for cancer. Preferably I would like to find a way that is repeatable — how cool would that be? — and I think, 'Is that too much to ask?' From where I'm sitting, it's not too much to ask, and it has become really important that I believe it is possible. It is like wanting the Nobel Prize: this isn't small, I want something really big. But it's not really Donna that wants it — I am trying to get my ego out of the way so the universe can channel information through me. Yes, my life can be saved for a period of time, but perhaps I've been put in this position where I can crack this code. Why not? I just can't think of any other use for me having cancer.

Michael Barnes

Life is very random. I am highly thankful that my cancer was caught in time but I don't ascribe that to some grand plan; I think I was enormously lucky. I don't think God 'acts' in that sense of action … So there's been a deepening in my sense of the randomness of life and my gratitude for life.

There was no particular reason for the Reverend Michael Barnes to be concerned when he had a PSA blood test done in 2004. For him, it was a piece of housekeeping as he moved to take on the role as minister at Crows Nest Uniting Church in Sydney. With no symptoms of serious illness, the news that he had prostate cancer and needed immediate surgery came as a bolt from the blue.

MICHAEL BARNES: When I got the diagnosis my first thought was something like, 'Bloody hell, I can't believe it.' My father had prostate cancer — he had died, though not from prostate cancer — so I was conscious that I needed to be a bit more careful. So when my PSA came back slightly high, I assumed that it would be something minor and my GP would say, 'No you're fine, don't worry about it.' So when I heard, it actually was quite a shock.

My first marriage broke up at the beginning of 2003, and I do wonder what impact that had on me getting prostate cancer, though it can never be proved. In 2004 I started going out with someone else, who is now my wife, and her support during that whole process was just amazing. We'd only been going out six months when I was diagnosed and I had the surgery nine months after we started going out, so it was a pretty full-on engagement in the difficult reality of a partnership. I think if you can go through those things together, you are on a pretty good wicket.

Cancer has changed my perspective on life and death in two ways: one, that it could actually happen to me; and two, I would call it good luck that I got the PSA test done. I had no symptoms, I should make that quite clear, so it is both remarkable and scary that I had a life-threatening illness which did not manifest in any way that I was aware of. I'm not one of those people who God tapped on the shoulder and said, 'Have a PSA test'; however, it does make one wonder about the timing of it. The cancer was one millimetre from spreading, so there was one millimetre between my life and death, so to speak. I have a cousin in Melbourne who is older than me; he was diagnosed with prostate cancer recently and his cancer had actually spread by the time surgery happened. He is now undergoing hormone therapy and at one point it was looking extremely serious for him. It was only when that happened to him that I got rattled about what happened to me.

Maybe there is no easier way to have these realisations. It doesn't have to be cancer per se — any tragedy or crisis is going to cause you to start reflecting on life differently and I think you probably have to go through the experience to figure it. I do have a view — and this was an intellectual view but now it's become more a life view — that life is very random. I am highly thankful that my cancer was caught in time but I don't ascribe that to some grand plan; I think I was enormously lucky. I don't think God 'acts' in that sense of action. I think more that God is in us and we are in God and held in the divine, but I don't think God orchestrates things for us, for our benefit. If I thought that way I'd have to say, 'Well, He didn't act that way for my cousin' — which I find a horrendous way of thinking. So there's been a deepening in my sense of the randomness of life and my gratitude for life.

When you go into hospital and you are having surgery, your world narrows down to a fairly small place, but when you come back home it starts expanding again. Every six months I have to see the surgeon for a PSA check. It heightens my anxiety, but at the same time it is like revisiting the experience and the relief and the gratitude — it's okay, I'm still okay. I am very thankful for my surgeon's medical skills.

Death is something I've thought about a lot, even before this. I ultimately don't find the thought of death scary. Now having said that, if I was told I'm going to die in six months, I'd be all over the place. But in the end there is some sort of sense that no, it's okay.

Diana Davidson

Oh, we are all going to die; there are only two things that are certain — you pop out, go through God knows what, and you die. I've had a busy life. I am very much an 'on the go' person, and I have found I've had to let go.

First treated for breast cancer in 1996, actress Diana Davidson (who has graced our television screens in many popular series since the 1970s) was found to have advanced secondary cancer in her left lung and in her bones ten years later. Diana has an exuberant theatricality as she speaks about her life: expressive, spirited, gesturing widely. Her husband, Max, cares for her in their home near the foreshores of Sydney Harbour, where Diana takes pleasure in birds and flowers, music, chocolate and her cat purring on her lap.

DIANA DAVIDSON: I think everybody would find their own way [through cancer]. It is a very individual thing, how people react to anything serious. People who stop and look when there has been a tremendous train crash — they are confronted with their own mortality; if they are *in* the train crash, that is a different question again, but it still needs an adjustment. It depends a lot on the personality and the personal experience, the belief, the faith of the person to whom this catastrophe has occurred.

A lot of people say, 'I'm fighting this; it's not going to beat me'; if they are having chemo, they go through with what is called a 'positive attitude'. Well, a positive attitude isn't necessarily a denial of what is bad — and, of course, there are people full of real faith, in religion or God or whatever. Naturally, the responsibility for all our illnesses is inside ourselves, each individual. Last time I went to the oncologist I said, 'Won't I come in one day and you'll say you've gotten rid of this?' and she said, 'I think you'd better go on down the road to Mary MacKillop Place; they are looking for a miracle.'

I keep on going along; I'm stable at the moment, and some [medical] people are surprised I got on as well as I did. But then I had breast cancer before, ten years ago. I had my treatment and then [the medical professionals] said, 'You are free of cancer.' Then I got a cold and a pain in my ribs and I felt really sick and couldn't eat properly. Breathing became difficult and talking almost impossible. Friends asked my husband, 'What on earth's wrong with Diana? She doesn't seem able to talk — so unlike her!' They found I had four litres of fluid in my left lung and then they found it was secondary cancer in my lungs and in my bones. So that is my present condition. I don't know whether the aches I get are from rheumatism: I stopped having HRT [hormone replacement therapy], and I was taken off the oestrogen drugs, which dried up every nook and cranny and all the joints.

Bone cancer is very painful; the only thing they can do is chop things out — it's not a pleasant prospect. I am very lucky I have a husband who is looking after me. We've been together for over 50 years and we've got three children, who are attentive and supportive to me, and my grandsons, and I have a lot of friends. When I was first diagnosed, I had support from them and I had a lot of fun; it is wonderful when people come and support you. One friend of mine, Julie Hamilton, had breast cancer when I did and she used to ring me up and tell me what to expect.

The sort of cancer I had first time round had a 60 per cent success rate. I thought not so much that my life was going to end, but even with all the people in my life, I felt a sense of aloneness. I didn't feel as bad as that when I got the secondaries because I'm older and you have to get used to disappointment. In theatre you don't get every part you go for; I think that has a lot to do with my capacity for disappointment.

I've always enjoyed yoga, I've always done mind/body/spirit sorts of things. I feel there is another dimension. I think the Buddhist philosophy is wonderful and people need to practise contemplation; it used to be regarded as an important thing, but the mystical part has gone out of it. I think the wonders of chanting are extraordinary and I do think these techniques can be learned. For cancer sufferers, anybody who is going to die. Oh, we are all going to die; there are only two things that are certain — you pop out, go through God knows what, and you die. I've had a busy life. I am very much an 'on the go' person, and I have found I've had to let go. The acting world is a great world; I suspect showbiz people have a special sort of courage. 'The show must go on' — that is somehow an attitude of acceptance.

I think if I'd been younger, it would have been different. I've always had lumpy breasts, medically speaking; [many years ago] I had a couple of scares and then I had a larger lump. I went to this doctor and he said, 'You go home and prepare for the worst.' He said, 'I am putting you into The Scottish Hospital and making an appointment with a leading oncologist, and he'll have to see you at 8 a.m. because you have to be at the hospital by ten.' So I came home and I was shocked; I thought, 'What am I going to do? There are my children, my husband …'

I spent a sleepless night with my husband and he swore if I lost my breast he would love me forever, but I did feel terribly abandoned, I felt I'd been condemned. But I didn't have time to think of this or that, so I went to the hospital at eight in the morning and Max was with me. The doctor got a large syringe, put the needle in my lump and drew out two vials of amber fluid. He said, 'That's benign, you can go home.' My husband was trembling and the doctor himself embraced the two of us, it was really quite sweet. The reaction then was almost worse, because I was suddenly facing all these terrible things and then just as suddenly it's 'Go home and have a cup of tea.'

That first time, I had to prepare everybody, I'd kissed the children goodbye. At this stage of my life, I've experienced all sorts of things, I'm not in agony, I'm being looked after.

I said to the doctor that I don't want to go past 80. There are too many people going past that. I don't think old age is a glorious thing at all.

I would tell anyone to use meditation — but not everybody can do meditation. I've been doing it through yoga for years. You go into meditation, you can go straight into a place where there is nothing; when you focus on the technique, it's easy. But I wouldn't be able to give anybody the golden keys because everybody has to find their own.

Stephanie Dowrick

It is a precious thing to learn that you can somehow survive even the worst losses. You will be changed — absolutely. But you need not be diminished. Whatever happens to us — and something happens to all of us — we are changed whenever life is hard … The question always is, are we changed for the better?

Interfaith minister and author of a number of internationally bestselling books, including *Intimacy and Solitude*, *Choosing Happiness* and *Forgiveness & Other Acts of Love*, Stephanie Dowrick grapples with tough spiritual, psychological and ethical issues in her writing and teaching. Her interest in sadness and loss is more than theoretical: Stephanie lost her mother to cancer when she was just eight years old, and when her own children were young, she experienced breast cancer herself.

Stephanie Dowrick: Not everyone finds something positive in cancer. There isn't a recipe or formula. And we need to be careful even talking about 'positives' I think, because when people are feeling only fear or rage, or great sadness or loss, it can be an added burden that they haven't also turned into a hero or a saint overnight!

On the other hand, it is amazing how any major transition — and illness is certainly that — forces, absolutely forces you to reassess your life in an honest way, even if it is the last thing you want to do. You simply *have* to decide what's important and what isn't. Of course what can also happen is that after the crisis of illness has subsided, you go back to your old ways of being more careless about life — taking it for granted. That can easily happen and sometimes it takes yet another crisis to push us to reassess. But almost all the 'positives' will come out of that process of reassessment, noticing that you are not immortal, noticing that time is precious, noticing who and what really matters to you — and doing something about that.

Losing my mother to cancer when I was very young shaped my life utterly — not just losing her, but also losing sight of myself as a truly lovable person. I am sure that's how she saw me. I have been very fortunate eventually to get some understanding of compassion out of that double loss, and also a more general sorrow about the suffering that humans experience and even sometimes cause one another. But it has been a very complicated journey. And, to tell you the truth, I would rather be less compassionate, less insightful, less concerned, less anything — and to have had the chance to see my mother grow old. She lost her chance to live a normal life span with all the discoveries and experiences that allows. My sister and I lost the chance to know her through all but the very earliest stages of our lives. She died more than 50 years ago, at the age of 38. It is painfully young. My children and my sister's children have totally missed out on her love as a grandmother. The losses are incalculable.

My own experience [of cancer] was that the entire process is completely unknowable and unpredictable in advance. There is absolutely no way that I could have predicted how intensely private I would feel about my diagnosis, how desperate I was that no one outside my immediate family would know until I myself had time to come somewhat to grips with it. I think that was related to my old childhood thing of not being able to bear other people's pity in the face of my mother's illness and death.

Along with grief, for me, there were odd feelings of shame. I felt I had let my children down. I knew it was irrational but it was what I felt. None of that was a 'positive' in any conventional sense. It simply told me a lot about my own vulnerability, despite so many years of psychological work. I was also coping with the shock of cancer while a very close friend was dying and I was dealing with a hideous court case over which I seemed to have absolutely no control. That loss of control leads to awful feelings of unreality and it takes great strength of mind to remain stoic in the face of that. I did pray a lot, really a *lot*. I guess the greatest positive is that it confirmed for me that nothing matters more than our relationships with the people we love most — and with God, if that's relevant. If I ever thought about dying, I wasn't regretting unwritten books — even though I am intensely engaged with my writing and other work. I was focused only on the horror that my own children might be left without a mother, as I was. That was my biggest fear. It wasn't even a positive to discover that; I already knew it. But perhaps I recognised that life is a gift, good health is a gift, in an even deeper and more grateful way than ever before.

I also wrote my book, *Forgiveness & Other Acts of Love*, out of that time, and discovered how utterly essential it was to focus not on my fears, but on what would lift me up and keep me going. Actually that's my life's work — but in writing *Forgiveness* I came to understand it profoundly. Writing that book I sometimes felt so inadequate to the task, yet my persistence and need for understanding drove me on and it helped me so much to write it. It has helped so many people to read it also, thank heaven. So, yes, focusing on what will get you through despite — and especially in the face of — your fears; knowing that much of what we worry about is irrelevant; unflinching love for life and one's dearest people: what could be more positive?

Of course I also asked, 'Why me?' It does you no good, though! Cancer is multifactorial. Some may say it is 'destiny' — but I don't go with the idea that everything happens 'for a reason'. I don't believe we live in that kind of ordered universe! We have to try our best to pluck ... not 'reason' perhaps, but some eventual meaning out of events. I was under enormous stress at the time. That did not help. I have envied people whose lives are not so obviously shaped by illness and death. But I am also aware that I have learned to be extraordinarily grateful for what I do have, and especially for becoming a mother myself.

In *Choosing Happiness* I wrote that 'grief and sorrow are not "negative" feelings' ... I feel that strongly. It is a precious thing to learn that you can somehow survive even the worst losses. 'Survive' is a tough word. You will be changed — absolutely. But you need not be diminished. Whatever happens to us — and something happens to all of us — we are changed whenever life is hard and we have to *meet* that — not avoid it, not send it back! The question always is, are we changed for the better? That's where choice and consciousness come in. That's where wisdom comes in. We might find strengths we never knew we had, but again I want to emphasise that we need to be very wary indeed about bringing too much idealism and judgment in here. People can be very critical of themselves or judgmental about others when it comes to crisis and how people 'ought' to respond. I would say that it is crucial to meet any loss or sorrow with a great deal of gentleness, kindness and patience, as well as compassion. Discovering that's possible, bit by bit, is already life-changing.

I have had many things to deal with in my life. In fact, my own cancer was relatively minor compared to some other agonies and losses. They have all added up to make me the person I now am. But I am also created by my joys, beliefs, values, and what's gone well. They 'make' me, too!

Glenda Goding

Cancer has been horrible to me — but it's also been good to me in the way that I have grown to love my family more than I did before. It makes you grow ... It hasn't been all doom and gloom — there has been some fun along the way, but the end of the story is too short.

In 2002 Glenda Goding, then 48, was diagnosed with breast cancer and had a mastectomy. She lived in Nhulunbuy in the Northern Territory, so for three months she had to fly to Darwin for chemotherapy every three weeks, then she relocated to Brisbane for radiation treatment. After that she went back to Nhulunbuy and recommenced the travel to Darwin for further chemo. The treatment appeared to be successful, and Glenda moved on with life. Then, in 2006, she was diagnosed with secondary cancer throughout her body, including her lymph nodes, parts of her spine and her liver. Before her diagnosis in 2002, Glenda and her husband Peter were 'walking on different paths', and their marriage of 30 years was threatened. Since the diagnosis, however, they have become very close. They have three adult children: Alison, Brett and Callen. With Alison, Glenda started attending church regularly and became a Christian in 2006. In coming to know Christ, Glenda did what she was physically

and emotionally able to in her weakened state, praying and visiting her church's healing rooms, yet she yearned to go further.

GLENDA GODING: Over the past few years I have grown up. I'm 53 already, but I thought life was about partying. Not that I was a heavy drinker, but I was a drinker. We were in the Northern Territory — I was diagnosed in Darwin. In the Northern Territory [drinking's] what you do, unfortunately. I found out [life's] not about drinking champagne, it's about having family and doing the right thing. I just know my family has really kept us going. We've had a good time really, though not enough time. If I had another 20 years it would be okay.

The relationship between Peter and me has grown so much. I'm not sure I would have expected that but I am so glad it happened. I think that is the main thing cancer has done for me.

Alison has worked very hard to keep me in the Christian life. I'd like to be able to say I'm a fully blown Christian; I believe in it all but I just haven't been able to take that extra step. I'd love to be able to step over the line and be right there but I haven't quite made it.

I've done nearly everything I need to do; I have just got a few things to sort out. We've all talked to family and kids, that's done; we've had lots of family time which has been really nice, but there are a few cards and things I haven't written. I've tried to cover most things; I've been doing that for about six months now, sorting out my jewellery and things like that.

Writing the cards is probably my next project; I've got it half sorted out. I'm glad I've had the chance, really glad. I look at people who have been run over and think that would be easy because you wouldn't know about it, but it is much better to have the time with the kids and be able to do what I've done.

My only fears for the future are for Peter and for my kids. That's the hardest part, knowing you are not going to see your kids again. I've had them for a long time and I want to keep them … we've had good times with them, and they haven't got into trouble, they've been really good kids. I love seeing them. And I've got beautiful grandchildren: Ali has two little boys; they are beautiful. That's really hard — little Dylan, he's four; we are really close.

Cancer has been horrible to me — but it's also been good to me in the way that I have grown to love my family more than I did before. It makes you grow. Even the travel and visiting the hospital: when you go to have your treatment, everyone is so helpful and positive — you think you are going to see your friends each week. It hasn't been all doom and gloom — there has been some fun along the way, but the end of the story is too short.

Alison Bennett

Glenda Goding and her daughter Alison are best friends as well as mother and daughter: they see each other or speak on the phone every day. All the same, the two women have experienced

Glenda's journey in very different ways. Glenda has had the physical challenges of cancer to face, while Alison has taken hope and strength from her relationship with God.

ALISON BENNETT: I see the situation a bit differently [to Mum]. I don't see the cancer bringing us together, I see God bringing our family together through what cancer has done. It's a bit of a roller coaster: you go on a journey with your emotions and you feel strong most of the time, then you hit a hitch and take a few steps back. But again you keep pushing through.

I still strongly believe that this isn't the end — I don't believe that Mum's going to die from cancer. Lots of people think I'm in denial, but God's given me — and lots of people around her — a faith to believe that there's going to be a healing testimony through all this. From the day that she was diagnosed with secondary cancer, I've had this feeling. And it's definitely not from me, because I wanted to give up and just let her go so that she's not suffering any more. I hate seeing her suffer and I hate seeing her having disappointment come again and again and again. But I think she's here for a greater purpose than just to prepare for death; even in these days, there are things to be done and to experience. And as a family we don't really come together to grieve; we cry and talk and chat, but it's not to wait for her to pass on, it's to enjoy her company as a family.

I've been a Christian for nearly four years, and from the day I became a Christian I've been pretty full-on! But I've had times where I've just been crying, screaming, angry. Now I feel that my relationship with God's been strengthened and I really feel He's borne us through this. One day I was driving my car and I was feeling really sad — Mum was going into hospital — and I was just praying that God would be here with me. But I felt Him saying to me, 'I *am* here with you, otherwise you wouldn't be coping as you are. Do you want me to move away so that I can come back and you can pick up where you're at?' So I really know that He is looking after all of us.

Seeing what Mum is going through now, she has had a really hard time, but there were times when she would have chemo with really limited side effects in a way that other people have not been able to experience. She would drive herself to chemo and radiation, drive back, then we'd go shopping. Or we'd go play with the kids; she'd still look after my boys when I went to work for an hour or two. Even this last Thursday, she was really tired and I said, 'Maybe I should get someone else,' but I didn't want her to feel like she wasn't capable — so I brought them over, and on the Sunday she went into hospital.

The hospital staff really didn't think that she was going to get out of hospital at one stage. Even on the Sunday night, they tried to prepare us because they thought she was going to go. And she's still here, talking with us now. We could overlook it, but I believe these are all miracles leading up to something — or allowing us to spend more time with her. Her speech has come back; in hospital her speech was very disjointed and unclear, and now she's speaking and thinking. Often when I look at her, I think she could just get up and walk.

I look to the future as much as I need to look to the future. Whatever happens, I know that God will help me through, so I'm not scared. If Mum did happen to pass away, I would be sad; Mum and I have always been best friends — we're on the phone at least twice a day, if I'm not here. I would miss her, but I would know that she was in a much better place; in heaven she won't be in any pain or any grief. And she won't have that sense of losing us, because it's going to be the most perfect, wonderful place. Selfishly, I would miss her — but I'm not scared for myself, I'm sad. But I still believe that she's going to be around! I think it's okay; I think it's all going to be okay.

The week after Glenda and Alison completed their interviews, Alison sent this email: *'It is with great sadness that I have to write and let you know that Mum passed away on Monday night at 7.05. My best friend, my mum, my hero. I love her and I am going to miss her, but I know that she is now pain, fear, and treatment free with a perfect body and in the presence of our Heavenly Father.'*

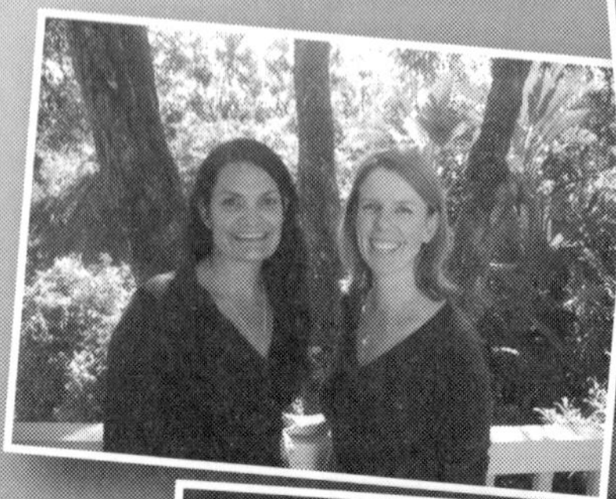
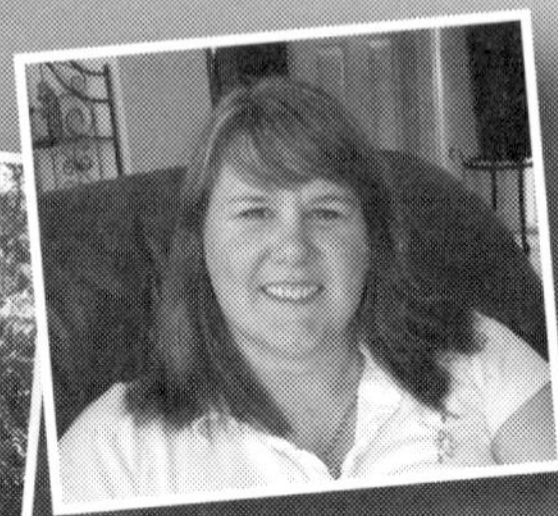
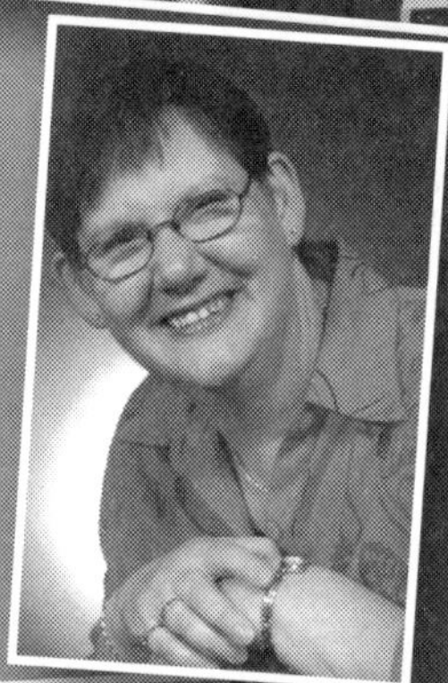
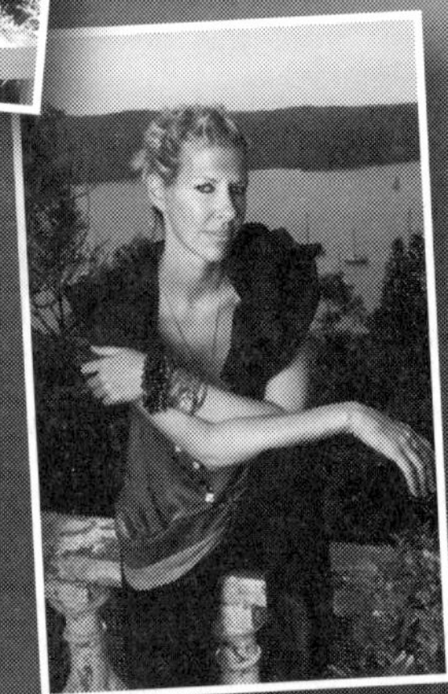
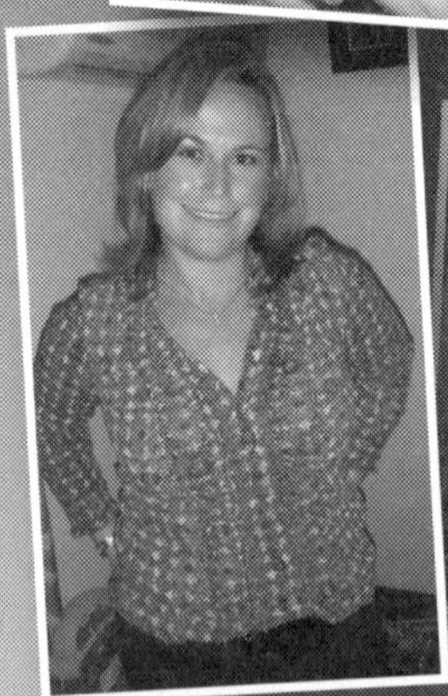
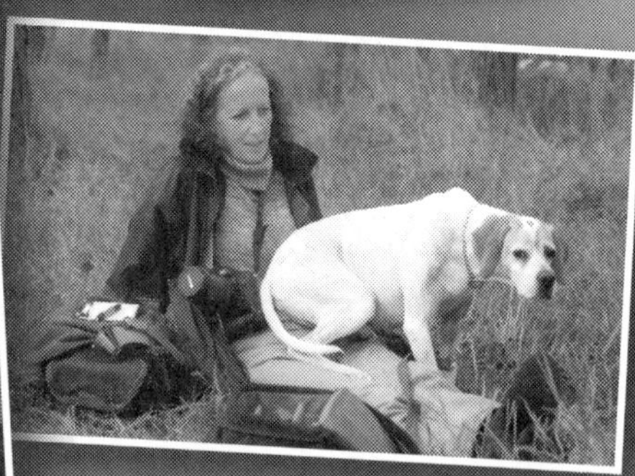

CHAPTER 4

A living legacy

> We will all die one day. That is one of the few things we can be sure of. But will we die well? That is less certain. Dying well means dying for others, making our lives fruitful for those we leave behind. The big question, therefore, is not, 'What can I still do in the years I have left to live?' but 'How can I prepare myself for my death so that my life can continue to bear fruit in the generations that will follow me?'
>
> **Henri J. M. Nouwen, *Bread for the Journey***

It would be wonderful to think that we could learn the major life lessons an easier way than by grappling with life-threatening illness. Listening to a great teacher, doing a course, reading a book (like this one). Certainly we can acquire 'head knowledge' that way, but it seems that 'heart knowledge' must be gained experientially. The cancer experience has the potential to change the texture, shape and resilience of our relationships, plant empathy deep inside us, prise open the generosity trapped in our hearts.

Sometimes we need an extreme experience to jolt us from the well-worn path we tread over and over. As Tony Burton put it after his lifelong friend, Ralph Jackson, died from a brain tumour, 'All too often we need — not just a tap on the shoulder, more like a smack in the head, wake up!'

One response might be to create a legacy for someone we have loved and lost. That legacy may be intimate and completely individual — like the children's book Tony wrote in honour of his friend — or it may be a shared experience. Ceremonies and events in the collective cancer landscape include everything from dragon boat races and CanTeen's national bandanna day to a Field of Women composed of 13,000 people in pink, or a lantern-floating ceremony on the Geelong waterfront. They are healing processes and rites of passage that prompt a time for reflection and connection.

For many of the sons and daughters in this book who lost their parents to cancer, there is a particularly strong sense of legacy. Even in the midst of dying, their mother or father showed them how to live, and they are determined to honour that memory in the way they live each day. Sandra Kent lost her mother to cancer before her three children were born, yet she has a sense that her mother is still with her as she finds her way as a parent herself. 'I can often hear her voice; I know she will always be with me.'

Heidi Middleton

> *You have a different level of compassion once you have been through something like cancer. I like to think I was compassionate and empathic before, but you can't go through this experience and not feel more for people in that situation — it connects you on a much deeper level.*

Sass & Bide designer Heidi Middleton was diagnosed with breast cancer in 2007, just 12 hours after she gave birth to her second daughter, Elke Bay. Even before her diagnosis, Heidi and her friend and business partner Sarah-Jane Clarke had been National Breast Cancer Foundation ambassadors for several years, supporting its campaigns with their profiles and their creativity.

HEIDI MIDDLETON: I went to the doctor for a pain in my breast not related to the cancer. I almost didn't go to the doctor — the pain went away in a few days anyway — but my husband insisted I go and have it seen by a GP. He didn't like the fact I had an infected sort of feeling in that breast while I was pregnant, so I went the same day to the hospital to have an ultrasound. Even the breast surgeon sent me home and said, 'You are right, it is nothing — just a blocked duct, anything more serious than that, like a cancer, would be painful; you have nothing to worry about.' But as I was walking out the door he said, 'As part of my practice I always get everybody to have a second ultrasound.' He'd confirmed there was nothing wrong so I left it six weeks; it was only at the insistence of my husband and mother-in-law that I went and had this follow-up ultrasound. The problem had gone away and everything was fine; I was about to have my baby. My husband did say I kept touching that breast; I didn't really notice it, but subconsciously I must have been a bit uncomfortable. When you are pregnant, your breasts are a bit tender anyway. So I went to the second ultrasound not worried about anything. They happened to find on the same breast in a completely different area a lump that didn't look good.

That was how it happened: my surgeon said if I had waited even just a few months, it probably would have been in my lymph nodes, which would have put me in a whole different situation. I definitely would have lost a breast; I managed to keep my breast. The lump was 1.7 centimetres, so it wasn't small but it wasn't large either, it was a good size. So I felt very blessed and lucky and fortunate. I feel like one of the luckiest ones: my prognosis is about as good as it gets, I think I'm down to a ten per cent chance it will come back. But I feel like I've gained so much from the experience, I've benefited from a bad situation with a happy ending. Not everyone is that lucky — a lot of people still live with the fear it might come back; for others it does come back or it gets them the first time. There are so many worse cases than mine. Even so, I had to go through the process of not knowing, thinking that I might be facing the worst. And that was my darkest time. All I thought about then was not seeing my daughters grow up; that was a feeling of pure dread. It was a dark, very sad feeling for about a week.

I've never felt fearful of death in regards to the final moment when you go. I just love life so much, I wish we could all live longer. I have never liked to dwell on the fact we all leave one day; I have such a hunger and thirst for life — I love it. This has made me know that I want to do the things I want to do while I'm here.

My diagnosis was certainly one of the most difficult experiences I've had in my life. But I think when you are in the moment like that and it's happening to you, you go into coping mechanism: one foot in front of the other and dealing with each situation as it presents itself. First and foremost I just couldn't believe how lucky I was to have the people I had around me. My husband and my first-born daughter were incredible; my mum and my mother-in-law were like guardian angels that descended upon us when they heard about all this. And the wonderful friends that I have were just an amazing source of inner strength during that whole intense few months.

One of my best friends was diagnosed two weeks before I was, and we were still in shock about that. Lucy kept saying to me, 'Are you angry yet?' — 'No, I'm not angry' — but not long after that I went through the different emotions. In retrospect, those emotions were quite clearly defined. I definitely was in denial in the beginning; even the night before I got my results, I slept well, I was absolutely 100 per cent sure there was no cancer. Then when I was diagnosed, it was disbelief and a bit of denial — 'This can't be happening' — and then I felt very angry and 'Why me?' It wasn't for a long period of time, only for a couple of days, but it was a very strong emotion. I did think I've been a good person, I've lived an honest life, a healthy life, I don't smoke, I don't drink heavily, I don't do drugs, I exercise — I was trying to think why it happened. After that I did feel quite depressed, especially before I had my results showing that my lymph nodes were clear — because there was a period of time when we weren't sure whether the cancer had spread to other parts of the body. And this was only just after I'd given birth, so the hormones were going crazy as well. So there was denial, anger, depression and then a feeling of acceptance — 'Okay, I've got it, for whatever reason I've got it, so let's work out how we are going to get through it.' I had to ask myself how I was going to carry myself through it emotionally: was I going to continue the anger, or feel sorry for myself, or was I going to try to see the humorous side of it.

I think by associating myself with the people that I did, they very much helped me have this attitude. I really did start thinking how lucky I was for so many reasons, and each morning I used to count all the reasons why I should be happy. And Lucy was two weeks ahead of me with chemo and radio and all that and also has young children; she was like this little beacon of light inspiring me to keep my chin up. On different days I remember feeling frustrated with the chemo; it is quite an isolating feeling, because it is so unique in its symptoms and the feeling you have. Even losing the hair — how many people lose their hair if they are not going through chemo? You do feel that even the people that love you so much can't quite relate to what you are experiencing. So I did form a very strong bond with people that were already friends but who were going through a similar experience; there was definitely that feeling of that connection where you just understand each other.

You don't want to judge people if they handle or approach your illness in a way you might not expect. There might be friends who you think might get in touch and they don't, and then there are people you might have met ten years ago who write you a beautiful letter. So you try not to judge, but I guess you do see people's true colours. The good and the positive that came from the love of friends is so much more overwhelming than anything negative that happened in that way. You see the strength in the people close to you as well; I was very much in love with my husband, but I feel even closer now; our bond is tighter and richer.

The cancer experience heightens those feelings that life is so precious and fragile and that we aren't invincible and we only have such a short space of time with the people that we love in our lives. It heightens the importance of telling those people that you love them — putting your thoughts into words rather than simply thinking them — and just expressing that love. I was probably a little bit that way anyway because I'm quite tactile and really do cherish and value those relationships, but I guess there has been a shift.

I guess you face your own mortality. It is the same as when you get sick; when you are coming out of it you think, 'Thank God that is over, I am lucky to be healthy again and to feel good.' But it is intensified when you get cancer; it is a very genuine threat to your life.

I've always considered myself more spiritual than religious; I have Christian values but I don't follow one belief. I don't know whether we go somewhere after life on Earth as we know it, but I do believe strongly in karma, that you get back what you give out in life. I've always felt that kindness is one of the most underrated virtues, and you should live your life in an honest way.

Things I was contemplating, I am now really addressing. I've had a strong interest in children's welfare from a very young age, and we are in the process of setting up a children's charity at the moment, through work. I've worked quite a lot with disadvantaged children in the past through Barnardo's and other organisations. But this has made me want to fast-track that and get it up and running, and not just talk about it for another couple of years.

You have a different level of compassion once you have been through something like cancer. I like to think I was compassionate and empathic before, but you can't go through this experience and not feel more for people in that situation — it connects you on a much deeper level. So all of that is another blessing, and it is a privilege to have gone through that. I don't think I could go through this and not want to help [other people with breast cancer]. But I didn't want it to take away from what I always wanted to do with children either — helping abused, disadvantaged children in general, children who aren't really exposed to love and care.

It is quite remarkable the strength you feel after going through something like cancer. Even though it was hard and challenging and scary, you do feel proud of having accomplished the treatment and got through that process while maintaining some dignity and humour and pride. It is a powerful feeling — though not in an arrogant way. Feeling clarity, being a bit more decisive about things. Not harsher, but deciding who you want to be around and who you don't and how you want to live your life. It is a great feeling; it is sort of breathed into you.

You get text messages and letters and things saying, 'You are so brave.' I kept thinking, 'This is not brave', this is happening for me and I'm getting through it the best I can. I would use the term 'bravery' in a different context. I think of a knight in shining armour; you *choose* to be brave, but for me — what other choice do you have but to go through the process? And I think most people would face it in a similar way.

What helped me might not help the next person, because we are all wired so differently. It was easier for me to look on the bright side and to look at the luck surrounding my situation. My prognosis was not as terrifying as it could have been, but I found trying to see the humour in it helped. Lucy and I did laugh our way through chemo; we'd pick each other up on different days. If you are not going to laugh, you'll cry, and you can get into that for days if you are not able to pull yourself out of it.

To try to maintain a sense of humour, and find people who are a bit lighter in spirit, and not dwell on the negative — that was something that helped me through. I refer to the chemo a lot because that six months was probably the hardest part of the treatment; I guess the fight comes out in you. So the whole time, through different ways, I was trying to stay on top of it — whether it was my humour, or putting a bit of bronzer on my face, or changing my scarf each day to make myself feel better, or painting my nails fluoro pink. Whatever it was, I would try each day, because you'd think you were on top of it and it would strip another layer back. I would get heartburn or my eyes would sting the whole time, so it felt better to keep them shut than open. The whole time it was a challenge but one you want to rise to because you think, 'I'm not going to let this thing take me right back down.'

I'd try to think of ways to keep my spirits up; I did think of the chemo treatments as laps under water, and the whole thing was a race. The chemo was the lap under water and you'd hold your breath and you'd get to the end and then you'd go again.

Liz Stone & Sharon Tregoning

LIZ: *Some relationships are stronger than ever, stronger than I ever dared dream of … Some of the delights have been some really grouse conversations with Sharon … the conversations become more authentic.*

SHARON: *The connection now is just mind-blowing … yet it is a double-edged sword: I am now enjoying this beautiful relationship I treasure but it is going to make losing her doubly hard.*

In 2003, Liz Stone was told she had breast cancer; it subsequently progressed to her lungs. She and her sister, Sharon Tregoning, discovered a significant history of cancer through their father's side of the family. As a result, Sharon has decided to have both breasts removed and reconstructed. Sharon is also setting up the Journey Beyond Cancer non-profit organisation to provide empowering services to adults who have had cancer — including massage, personal training and financial advice — to help them regain some 'normality' in their lives.

LIZ: When I first had breast cancer it was, by my choice, a fairly solitary journey; I took a year off work and did all the treatment. The second time, I went to the oncologist and she said, 'You have spots on your lungs.' I got home and rang one of my closest friends and he said, 'How does this impact on your spiritual journey?' and I said, 'The reality is it makes no difference at all in terms of the spiritual journey,' which to me has always been a lot more important than the physical.

Spirituality has always been really important to me. It changed dramatically at the end of 2004; I left a mainstream Christian church and I now belong to a Spiritualist church. I am at peace and very happy with the Spiritualist philosophy of life. Spiritualism holds that there is more to life than this physical body, this physical experience. The physical body is a vehicle that allows me to enjoy here and now, and I have a spirit that lives forever, that always continues to evolve. While my body may cease to live, my spirit will always live. Death has never been something I was uncomfortable with; I believe in honouring people and that whole process of death and funerals is a huge chance to do that and to help families move on.

As with everything in life, there has been a variety of responses from people. Some relationships are stronger than ever, stronger than I ever dared dream of. I feel blessed to have had the opportunity to know that I am loved. People have made all sorts of wonderful offers of help. Earlier this year, a group of family and friends came and helped finish the makeover of my backyard. But in spite of all the offers of help, it's also difficult because I'm fairly independent and believe in doing things while I can. At present I don't need a lot of practical or physical support, I am still quite able to look after myself. I find that I feel most supported by those who see me as living with cancer rather than dying from cancer. I have a really good life. I can take an hour over breakfast if I want to and it's okay because there is nothing else I need to be doing.

Some of the delights have been some really grouse conversations with Sharon. It was her birthday recently and she wanted to go somewhere for her birthday for lunch, and I knew that if we booked to go there, I wasn't going to physically make it. Once upon a time I would have said, 'Oh, yeah,' and then rung up on the day and said, 'I'm not well, I'm not going.' But now it became, 'I don't want to hurt you, this is where I am.' So the conversations become more authentic. And I don't leave stuff undone like I would have, which gets a bit in people's faces but that's me: welcome to my journey.

SHARON: Liz is the eldest, I'm the youngest, and there is a significant age gap in between. We haven't been all that close; we've been through different journeys and phases and so forth. My hubby and I started on a journey of self-awareness and a change in spirituality this year, and it is partly through this that we now have this unbelievable relationship. I'd sort of packaged where I was at: 'I am losing my sister but what am I grieving about because we didn't really have a relationship?' I thought, 'I'd like to have a close relationship but it might not be her priority, she is the one with limited time here,' but now this is what I want, this is what she wants. The connection now is just mind-blowing; some of the conversations are — some would say macabre, but they are honest. I don't see it as a sisterly bond — Liz is someone who is really important in my life. So that for me has been the best thing to come out of it, yet it is a double-edged sword: I am now enjoying this beautiful relationship I treasure but it is going to make losing her doubly hard, and that really bites. I try not to focus on that, I try to enjoy what we've got, particularly while she is so well at the moment. But every now and then it bites hard. After Liz was advised of the diagnosis, I didn't react very well. I automatically thought, 'Okay, my sister has breast cancer, what does that mean for me?' It was pretty selfish, the way I reacted.

Liz got in touch with Dad's sister and found out [cancer] is rife through Dad's side of the family: four generations. There was a huge split on Dad's side of the family so we didn't know any of this until three years ago. That set a whole different chain of events into action. Liz underwent gene testing, but they weren't able to identify the gene; I know at the time it was really good for her but for me it was useless, because I couldn't be tested. If they'd found the gene it was a 'no brainer', the boobs were coming off, but this decision is a whole lot harder. I have a 30 to 40 per cent chance of developing cancer, and while the numbers are in my favour, [having my breasts removed] is a hugely emotive decision.

I am a person who likes caring and helping people, so I said to Liz, 'Is there anything that would have made it easier?' and she said, 'To be touched in a non-medical massage would have been lovely,' and [the idea of the foundation] just expanded from there. We've been trying to sell our business for the last two years; we think we are very close, but I can't focus on Journey Beyond Cancer until I've got that happening, so that's the next step for me. Yes, it is about honouring Liz, but it is not defining her by it, it is about bringing something good out of something pretty crappy and wanting to help people and make a difference in their lives. The services we offer will empower them with some control when they could be out of control. I've got very grand plans for it; sometimes it is really daunting, but I keep coming back to the base of what I want to do and why I want to do it — helping people to live the life they want.

LIZ: I have a 23-year-old with a severe intellectual disability who operates at the level of a two-year-old, so I've had a fair degree of difficulty in terms of raising children and having to be assertive and an advocate and all sorts of things, doing things I'd never dreamed I would. All of that still wasn't sufficient to bring about these changes in my life. You know how you get some kids who are determined to learn things the easy way and some do it the not-so-easy way? I think I might put my hand up to say I'm a bit out there ... There are some ways you learn things better than others.

Liz Stone passed away on 3 February 2007, four months after this interview took place.

Mike Schram

Elaine looked, at the end, like a starving child. She couldn't walk, feed herself, wash, sit on the toilet; she had no hair … The fact is, though, that when someone is stripped of these things we see them as the pure, beautiful soul they are. I never loved Elaine more than when she needed me to be there for her only. All I lived for was that I could help, and so I (so I'm told) was the best nurse she could have. I do hope so. I tried so very hard for the person I loved.

Mike and his wife, Elaine, were partners in the truest sense of the word. Married for just over 20 years, together they ran Shoot Photographic in Campbellville, Ontario, specialising in horse photography. Their work was both seasonal and intense: spring and summer brought back-to-back horse shows, while winter was a time to dig in and catch up on business and home life. In 20 years of marriage, they spent only three weeks apart. Elaine died of ovarian cancer on Valentine's Day 2007.

Mike Schram: Cancer is really difficult on anybody but Elaine is in a better place — that is the only way I can look at it. For me, I miss my cuddles and I'm lonely but that is really the downside for me — I figure she is better off now. I have no idea where she is, mind you, but I have to believe that all the cares and worries that go on here, are not there where she is now. As long as you are alive in this world you've got to keep going and make do with the best of what you've got, and make a good life for yourself and try to make a good life for everybody else. For the last year, my entire goal was keeping her alive, making things the best I could for her, and I think I did that. I certainly worked hard at it. So now I've got to do the best I can and keep going for myself.

As a caregiver (the person who is as close as possible to the 'patient') who has to deal with the continuing degeneration of the 'patient' (loved one), you see that the 'patient' is stripped of all worldly blessings. Elaine looked, at the end, like a starving child. She couldn't walk, feed herself, wash, sit on the toilet; she had no hair ... The fact is, though, that when someone is stripped of these things we see them as the pure, beautiful soul they are. I never loved Elaine more than when she needed me to be there for her only. All I lived for was that I could help, and so I (so I'm told) was the best nurse she could have. I do hope so. I tried so very hard for the person I loved.

We were married just over 20 years and knew each other for 23. There was a week-long Arabian show that was held in Saskatchewan that Elaine photographed by herself for three years running, and those three weeks were the only time we were apart the whole time we were married, otherwise day and night we were together all the time. It was like being married for 40 years, but that was what we wanted and we wouldn't have it any other way.

After the winter was over [following Elaine's death] I didn't know if I had to reinvent myself to make a living, or what everybody was going to be like. [At the horse shows] I tended to flit around three or four rings and pick up bits and pieces, and she stuck in a couple of rings and visited everybody. She was the heart and soul as far as the company was concerned; she would talk to everybody, and I'm not that way inclined, I'm not a really gregarious kind of person.

There were over 150 people at the funeral, and I think over 100 of them were the horse community — they came from everywhere. The next show I photographed was three weeks after she died. It was a show I normally did myself; I went on Saturday and everybody looked at me funny and I went on Sunday and got offered five new shows — people were just rallying around. When I got to the first 'A' show, they were coming up to me left, right and centre. That first show was really hard. I always find condolences hard, partly because some don't know how to do it, some don't do it at all, and it reminds you every time.

[In that community] four or five are widows, I'm the only widower. We've all lost our partners to cancer so we have a little club, we compare notes and help each other out. It is a very insular community, but once you've proven yourself, they won't let you down at all. You can't let anybody else down, either, it is give and take.

And I had a dog nobody would take. Billie was Elaine's dog, glued to her; she didn't come near me for about eight months or more when we first adopted her. I told one of my good friends I still had the dog. She said, 'What do you still have the dog for? That is the worst thing you can do for the dog — she is expecting to find Elaine everywhere she goes, she doesn't like you in the first place, she should be taken someplace that is totally foreign to her so she can start her life over again — which is what everybody has to do.' Anyway at the beginning of July finally the dog was taken away. The dog is really happy now, she is on a farm with four other dogs, she is having a great time.

It's kind of funny because I was really waiting to become 50 years old. My dad was the oldest of the men of my family when he had his first heart attack at 49; he had ten more before he died when he was 59. So I had that staring me in my face, and my mum's side of the family had cancer and strokes. So hitting 50 was really great. It had always been in the back of my mind that Elaine would probably have to do without me. Elaine's family never had cancer on either side and she is the youngest. So all the rules are out the door for both of us. We were looking at her having to deal with things without me, so all the life insurance was the other way around: she would be well provided for if I went, and we had just enough so I could pay off a few things and hope for the best if she went, which is what is happening.

I haven't had a reduction in the number of shows I was going to do for the year. When I told them, 'I don't know what to do because it's only me and I'm not going to hire somebody to hold the camera and look like they are doing a job and turn out rotten pictures,' the show managers have gone, 'It's you we want doing the shows; whatever you can do, come and do the shows.'

So I've had multi-ring shows, I've been run off my feet. It is holiday time here, bills coming in, got shingles, but you go in every day. And today I had a load of faxes down onto the floor and I had people come in and write me a couple hundred dollar cheques. So as far as I'm concerned everything is bright; I still don't get a cuddle in the morning but everything is bright. Every day is an adventure, there's no two ways about it. Every day is an adventure so grab it for the adventure, and if you get beaten down, shake your head and get back up again.

Tony Burton

All too often we need not just a tap on the shoulder, more like a smack in the head: 'Wake up!' ... You must be conscious and you must be aware even of the smallest experience and you must have a sense of gratitude for what you are going through, all the small, small things that you experience each day.

Tony Burton is a Perth-based lawyer. After his initial intense grief over the death of his childhood friend, Ralph Jackson, Tony found instances of serendipity that enabled him to turn his

sorrow into compassion and empathy. He also found concrete ways of making beautiful things that would convey a sense of the heart and soul of his lifelong friend.

TONY BURTON: I'd known Ralph for a very long time. I'd grown up with him, been to primary school and high school with him, and we kept in touch when we did our respective university degrees. He had been working over in the US; when he returned to Sydney, I was living in Perth, so in terms of day-to-day contact there wasn't much, but there was a very strong bond. The impact his illness, then his death, had on me was not what I had expected. I didn't expect to be as shaken up as I was. I was just overwhelmed and I was having enormous difficulty dealing with the fact of his death.

The immediate issue was coming over to Sydney to spend some time with his family and to be involved in the funeral. I'm a shy person; I don't normally speak much unless I have to. Ralph's sister, Belinda, had contacted me to ask if I'd prepare some music to be played for the funeral. I thought, 'Good, I know Ralph's mind, I know what he'd like', so that was a nice contribution to make. I was working away on that and a few days later she rang up and said, 'We'd also like you to do one of the eulogies', at which point I froze with fear. I thought, 'This is something I've got to do,' but it was overwhelming. I found myself lying awake at nights and getting increasingly stressed and worked up as to what I could do.

This is going to sound very bizarre, but I consulted a kinesiologist. I'd go running along the beach of a weekend and I used to see this queue outside a doorway; I thought it must be an outlet selling tickets to a show or a bakery or something. I walked past to try to find out what was going on, and people were queuing to see this guy. I'd heard about him being a good person to speak to, so on the Saturday before the funeral I went and saw him. I was in a terrible state, and he just looked at me and said, 'This is very serious, what's going on? You have a severe emotional block.' At which point I broke down in tears and he asked me what had happened. I explained and he said, 'You've lost a true friend. You don't have that experience very often in your life, that you have a true friend.' He said this is very serious but also that it is easy to deal with. I told him, 'I've got to go to the funeral, it's really important to me but I haven't got the energy.' He talked me through it; he said, 'The eulogy, what is it all about?' I ended up saying, 'Look, I shouldn't be talking to other people, I should be talking to Ralph,' and he said, 'That is what you do, write him a letter.' And from that moment on it unfolded. I went straight home and started writing this letter. I didn't want to talk to people and say, 'Ralph was this, that and the other,' I wanted to speak to Ralph to say, 'I am missing you, and this is what I'm thinking about.'

It was almost like the universe touched me, and all this stuff opened up. I arrived at the airport to fly over, thinking, 'I haven't got enough head space for this.' I checked in and straight away they put me at the front of the plane on my own, which was great. What I really wanted to do while I was in Sydney was spend some time with Ralph's daughters, his wife, his mother, and with his sister, Belinda, as well. Over the next 24 hours, everything just fell into place; someone would say, 'Can you look after the girls? We've got to go pick up the order of service.' Then they'd say, 'Can you stay with Sheila [Ralph's mother]?' I ended up being able to spend time one on one with each of the people I wanted to connect with.

It felt as if I'd been touched by something special. After the funeral, when we were back at Ralph and Sally's house, I was able to talk to kids I didn't know and play games with them and get them laughing. I got to talk to different people — I just felt as if I was doing something really good; it was almost as if I was being directed to offer comfort.

Shortly before I flew over for the funeral, my son said to me, 'What's your favourite word?' — it was one of those kid questions — and I said, 'I like the word serendipity.' I got on the plane to fly back, and it was the same kind of good fortune as when I checked in. This time, they'd issued the boarding pass and the guy looked at me, took the boarding pass out of my hand, tore it and put me up the front of the plane alone. I sat on the plane, opened up a book and the first chapter I opened up, on the first page, they started talking about serendipity. As I talk about it now it sounds nutty, but it was very real. There was a whole series of these things that happened; it burned brightly for a couple of weeks.

I was trying to find some meaning or purpose, or something I could do to help Sally and the girls. From the other side of the country it is really hard, there is only so much you can say over the phone — they are in a really raw place, you want to help, you want them to rebuild. One morning I started writing a story. It was intended as a story that draws children towards focusing on positive emotions and happy experiences and it directs them towards sharing them with parents or whoever is reading with them. It was also strongly inspired by Ralph. One of the other people who spoke at the funeral was a university friend and he told this story. Ralph apparently had a fan club of a few young women who would hang around him; one girl once said, 'Ralph — that's a really strange name. What's it short for?' He shot back with 'Ralphred'. So the first line of the book is, 'Have you seen the Ralphreds?' The Ralphreds are watching and listening but they'll only come if you are doing the right thing and if you are focusing on the right things.

The process of writing the book became a very therapeutic experience because I was doing something that could make a contribution, and getting people around me involved helped me connect with them. Christine, a woman I work with, has always adorned her office with artwork done by one of her daughters. I knew the daughter was either finishing high school or had just finished so I said to Christine, 'Can I speak to your daughter? I have a proposal for her.' She probably thought I was from another planet originally. I gave her the text and said, 'You just do what you think is right and come up with some pictures.' So I got her involved, then I got my daughter involved: she helped me out with words and font and text, and different images. After it was written and the images were combined with the text and we found the right paper to put it on, we found some special paper and silver leather for the cover and had it bound up. I wanted to present it so it would have an impact, so I got my kids to help me and we found a big box, painted it up and stuck fairy stones, coloured glass and stars on it. Initially I thought I'd just send it out of the blue, anonymously, but I thought it might have been a bit upsetting so I brought it over to Sydney in person. I remember giving it to Belinda; we were at a café in Bondi. I wanted to know if she thought it would be okay to give to Ralph's family. She wandered off and sat down on the grass and read the book. She came back with tears in her eyes, but they were good tears. The same thing happened when I gave it to Sally; I realised it had touched them.

I was very conscious of trying to do something that felt authentic. I could have just given a big donation or sent flowers, but that wouldn't have done any real good. The experience also got me thinking about proper gifts. Now at Christmas time or on my birthday I say to my kids, 'Please don't buy something for me.' So every Christmas and birthday there is a short story, a poem, a picture — something they have done — and I sit with them and either read the story or go through the poem, and I keep them in a volume of my treasures.

Ralph's death has made me conscious that we drift in a very unfocused way through life without stopping and asking, 'Why are we doing this? What is the reason for this?' — all these conventions we comply with. Maybe it caused me to think a little more about things and to seek some purpose and meaning. I'm not sure I'm getting it yet, but at least I'm asking the questions.

All too often we need not just a tap on the shoulder, more like a smack in the head: 'Wake up!' There's a quote from Warren Zevon, the musician, who died a few years ago. He was on the David Letterman show and was asked one of those stupid questions that people ask in interviews. Letterman said, 'Do you have any advice?' And Warren Zevon said, 'Enjoy every sandwich.' At one level, it is trivial, but at another level, it is really profound. You must be conscious and you must be aware even of the smallest experience and you must have a sense of gratitude for what you are going through, all the small, small things that you experience each day.

Sandra Kent

I was going to do everything the conventional way, but that way has never really suited me, so it took this to discover who I was.

When her mother was diagnosed with oesophageal cancer, Sandra gave up the good life as a single banking professional in

Sydney to be with her mother in Johannesburg. Her mother died in 2003. Now married with two children and living in Perth, Sandra believes that her new life would never have been possible had it not been for her mother's illness. In an email, Sandra wrote, 'I needed something to alter my course as I was on a path to destruction; I probably would have had a fatal car crash or something similar by now.'

SANDRA KENT: I'd booked Mum a ticket to come and live with me in Sydney. She never boarded that flight because she was diagnosed with cancer two weeks after I booked the ticket. I heard she had had problems with her throat for a few months and, next minute, she was diagnosed with oesophageal cancer. That was the Wednesday; by the Friday I had booked a flight and I landed in Johannesburg and headed for [my sister] Lyndsay's place, where Mum was living. On the Monday, Mum went in for a major operation to remove the tumours in her throat. I spent the next month with her while she went through 14 days in intensive care and another month in hospital.

I had been living the life of Riley in Sydney. I was sailing every Saturday and Wednesday, I had a great social life, I drove a nice car, I had everything going for me. I had a really nice life and I was taken away from that and put into a very hostile, sterile hospital environment for a month. But it brought home to me that our life is so fragile. I would walk along the ward every day praying for all the sick people in it; being there really inspired me to have compassion.

When I returned to Sydney from South Africa, I went through a major transition. I was quite senior in my church and used to run the hospitality room; I was a committed Christian; I didn't drink too much, I was on a good spiritual path — but when I got back from South Africa everything just went haywire. I got very rebellious and angry. I started drinking a lot and got onto a very reckless path. I would go to the pub by myself, not care who I was talking to — I was doing things that were very out of character. I think a lot of it was me trying to stop myself from thinking about my mum, who was at this stage going through chemo to try to get rid of the cancer. I guess it was a denial phase because I didn't want to face up to what was happening; but at the same time I was very content with my own company. I'd been single for a long time and I was starting to enjoy myself — coming into my own, doing what I wanted to do.

If it hadn't been for Mum's illness, I think I would have carried on going to church three times a weekend, waiting for that lovely Christian man to pluck me out of the hospitality room and do the right thing, then carry on living the life that I thought was there for me. I thought that was it, you know — I was going to do everything the conventional way. But that way has never really suited me, so it took this experience with Mum to discover who I was.

In May a year later, my sister phoned me and said the doctor didn't think Mum had long to go: she was on a downward spiral. So I hopped on a plane, saw how bad Mum was, went for a job interview, got the job, flew back to

Sydney, packed up, and within five weeks was back there, without even thinking of what I was giving up. I thought Mum was going to get better, and I'd go there, and she could live with me in Jo'burg; I could take care of her, and we could have a cushy life. I left a very good job at a merchant bank; I think I might have already jeopardised my career in the banking sphere because I had been so preoccupied with what was going on with my mum, so it was probably a good time for me to get out of that environment before I completely threw the game away.

When I got back to South Africa, I went to visit my mum, and she had deteriorated and was in excruciating pain. That was in July. My mum passed away on 14 September; she went downhill quickly and ended up in a hospice. The cancer went to her brain: she just couldn't balance any more, she kept falling and really damaging herself, so we decided the hospice was the safest place for her. The doctor had phoned me and said I'd better get down there. She was in Durban at that stage, 600 kilometres away, so I picked my uncle up and we drove the 600 kilometres. When we saw her, the death rattle had started, and I told her she should go and have peace and not hold on any longer. We had a very strong bond — my mum was my best friend, she was the person I told everything to, she'd always been there for me. It was at 2 a.m. the next morning I kissed her on the forehead and she took her last breath.

I have no regrets. I am so pleased I gave up everything cushy to go to horrible, dangerous Jo'burg with nothing, so I could say goodbye to her. In a way it's released me; I'm free. [After that] I wasn't trying to live for my mum any more and I wasn't trying to live through her illness. Every decision I made was for me; it wasn't whether it would suit her or fit in with her chemo. It was a very big weight lifted off my shoulders. Also I knew she was at peace, I knew she was with God and He was holding her, and she wasn't in pain any more. She had been in difficult personal circumstances. She had lost everything, she didn't really have anything any more. She was always worrying about where she was going to work — a week before she died she said to me, 'Where am I going to get a job?' — you'd think that for somebody so ill, it would be the last thing on their mind. She had been in so much pain and stress, so it was a big comfort to know she had gone and had peace.

[Before my mum's illness] I'd thought my calling was spiritual healing. I'd lay on my hands — I really thought this was it — I couldn't even save my own mum. After my mum died I became very despondent about the healing side of spirituality; I was angry that God hadn't used me to heal my mum. Eventually, it made me realise it is not up to us who He heals. It was a big wake-up call spiritually; I still pray for healing and I know God heals. With my children, if they hurt themselves I pray for healing and every time they heal quickly, I thank God. It has just deepened my respect and love for Him. I'm a bit of a control freak — sometimes it is actually reassuring that we are not in control. This has made me relax into God more, it has made me surrender more to Him rather than try to be a soldier all the time.

These days, when bad things happen to people I am more philosophical about it. I always thought I wasn't a sympathetic or empathetic person, I always felt I was quite cold. I don't suffer fools, I'm not a gusher, but as soon as I meet somebody who is going through it, the words and the comfort just come out. You know what they are going through and what they need, you know they don't need to be bombarded with falseness, you know they might need a meal made for them.

My sister, Lyndsay, is four years older than me. We'd always fought but we seem to have both taken the pain for my mum for each other. We are on the phone three times a week for an hour: the way I used to talk to my mum I now talk to my sister. This experience has definitely drawn us together; we have this sadness that we share.

I have Mum to thank for [my wonderful husband] Mark, too. If she hadn't gotten ill, I would never have gone back to Jo'burg, not in a million years, and I would have been waiting around the church hall for a Christian man. I met Mark in a pub called Billy the BUM'S, through a sailing friend. I so wasn't interested, I was still grieving my mum — the last thing on my mind was romance. Mark tried to court me for a month before I realised, and we ended up hitting it off; we actually kissed on my mum's birthday. We got engaged a couple of months later, got married and then fell pregnant.

When it comes to the big events like our wedding and our children being born, I do feel sad not to be able to share them with Mum but then an overriding peace comes in. I know Mum is at peace, I don't have to worry about her any more, so the peace I get from knowing that is stronger than the angst I have that she is not here. I often talk to her — that may not be correct in some Christian doctrines, but it gives me comfort. I'll be hanging out washing, all these little clothes, and I'll think, 'Wow, what was I like when I was a baby?' That is the one thing I'd like, to know if my kids are like I was, because only a mum remembers those things. I can often hear her voice; I know she will always be with me.

This experience has introduced me to death; I'm not scared of seeing a dead body now. I think of my mum lying there; she lay from two until seven in the morning before they came and took her away. It was just her body, not her soul, not her spirit — it was just a shell. I'm not afraid of death any more; I know what comes is going to be better than this life.

I haven't changed fundamentally, I've just grown up — I've become an adult. If life gets tough for me — and I am going through a tough phase with my dad having a serious illness now — I don't just look to have a glass of wine and a cigarette to calm me down, though I still enjoy my wine! Now I have a cup of tea and work through it. So it's helped me to not run away from my problems. I've watched my mum in the shower weighing next to nothing, I've held her in my arms, I've listened to her death rattle. I often have a reality check and say, 'Hang on, just because you've got two children that aren't going to sleep and you haven't cooked dinner yet, that is reality, it's not cancer.'

Deena Raphael & Lauren Adlam

> LAUREN: *Deena and I were talking about the motherless community … We came up with the idea that people could plant a tree in memory of their mums on Mother's Day and do something positive for her and give a purpose to the day.*
>
> DEENA: *The feedback we get from those who participate is positive and very touching. Trees for Mum has been very rewarding for me — it's a great feeling to share this with the community.*

Friends at work first of all, Deena and Lauren soon discovered they had something deeper in common: their mothers both died of cancer when they were young. Deena and Lauren also shared a desire to help other people who had lost their mothers, so in 2002 they set up Trees for Mum, a Mother's Day memorial tree-planting event. So far, more than 16,000 people have taken part in the Trees for Mum program.

DEENA: My mother died when I was 16, nearly 20 years ago. She was 43 and she had what started out as cervical cancer; it spread, and she ended up having it in her lymph nodes. She died ten months after she was diagnosed; she had surgery and chemo and radiation, and she sought lots of alternative treatments as well. There was my dad, my sister and I; my sister was 13, three years younger than me.

Lauren: For me, I was 21 when Mum died, and that is coming up to ten years ago this year. She had pancreatic cancer; similarly, it was less than a year from diagnosis when she died. I've got two older brothers and my dad, so I was in charge of the house from then on — which wasn't necessarily a bad thing, I quite enjoyed taking on that role. I had to grow up really quickly and I was at the age that it wasn't too early to grow up, either, so I relished the fact I was in charge and held the family together.

People look at me like I've got two heads when I say this, but I'm a better person because of what happened to me. Obviously I'd give anything to have Mum here and be sharing my child with her, and she never met my husband. Mum was an incredibly positive person, and I think I've become an incredibly positive person. She was all about living for the moment, not having fights with people and walking away, making the most of everything you've got. Whether I would have been like that too if she was still alive or not, who knows, but I definitely think I'm a more well-rounded person as a result of what happened. If someone says to me, 'You are like your mum,' that is the ultimate compliment because for me, she was the pinnacle of what I would like to be.

DEENA: For me the positives didn't come about as clearly. I felt very shocked that my mother died; my family didn't really prepare us. My dad and my mother chose to keep it — not secret, because we knew she was sick, but I was shocked that she died. That really came as a big blow; I didn't know how to handle that. I had one year of high school left then I went away to college. I had this new life living away from home, with new friends and a new environment and, in a way, that was how I dealt with it, but I missed Mum so much and I felt very lost without her.

After I graduated from college I wanted to travel. I thought I could go out and find myself. So for me, in the end, that was a real positive that came out of losing Mum — I travelled the world. I think she instilled that spirit in me; she encouraged me to be an exchange student and I went to France for a semester in high school. She never went overseas and she encouraged me to travel and I had that in my mind — I wanted to see the world because she never got to. I travelled for a year thinking I would eventually reach a destination that would 'fix' me. I saw many beautiful places and met kind, generous people and learned to be alone and quiet with my own company. I finally understood, 'Wherever you go, there you are' — you can't get away from yourself. I began to accept myself.

LAUREN: My situation was very different to Deena's because Mum very much kept me in the process throughout her death: she planned her own funeral, she wrote a message for everyone to read. Obviously you never truly get a chance to say goodbye, there are always things you want to say, but we managed to start processing it before it happened, so I think that made a difference to me as well. I thought it would be really confronting to see her after she died, but it wasn't, it was kind of peaceful. So from that point of view, I guess death is a bit less scary. I gratefully believe that wherever she is, she is very much part of our life; she can see what we are doing. That is almost unnerving sometimes, but I look forward to making her proud of whatever she can see.

DEENA: Maybe death is not as scary to a certain degree because I've known someone who has died. But that said, since having children I've developed a new fear of dying as it relates to leaving my children. Losing my mother has had such a lasting impact on me; the thought of them having to experience that sort of loss is unbearable. If my daughter says, 'Don't go, I need you,' I hear, 'Don't die, I need you,' as opposed to 'Don't go to the shops, I need you.' I know it's an irrational fear, and it can be exhausting.

LAUREN: People in similar situations expect you to know what they are going through because you've been through it yourself, but I find the exact opposite. Everyone's situation is unique. Some people aren't close to their mums and their mum dies, and so then they have to deal with the whole grief of the loss of the relationship they never had. My relationship with Mum was unique, so I know what *I* went through. I found it a little bit frustrating when people would say, 'I know what you are going through,' and I'd think, 'No, you don't, you've got no idea.' Some very close friends of mine have lost their mums as well and so I am very conscious of saying, 'It's different for you.' A lot of that has come out of Deena and me discussing our stories, because we have very different stories and different ways things have happened to both of us.

DEENA: I think I still struggle with what the right thing to say is. I don't have the magic answer. I feel I should know what to say, but I don't. But I still feel I have this connection to other people who have lost their mother. While you don't necessarily know what they are going through, I definitely feel this empathy. It is very emotional and a very powerful loss, especially for young people. For most people, their mother is a very significant person in their life. Even if the relationship is bad, she is the person who made you; there is so much around that. Losing a parent can be a time to reflect at any age, but it really shapes you when it happens to you in your formative years.

LAUREN: I guess you can still make your mum proud, even though she is not here; that is something that is very important to me. I would like to think wherever she is, she can see me and think, 'She's doing a good job.' I think how much she would love her grandson. She never saw any of her grandchildren, never saw any of us get married or anything like that. Obviously you think of the opportunities that are lost, but I talk about her as part of my life, because she *is* part of my life. I don't have memories and think, 'You can't say that because that is the past' — there are some really positive memories. I am conscious about not talking too much about the old times in front of Dad's current wife, because she is very much part of our family now as well. She understands it is important to us.

DEENA: For me, the loss was a long time ago, more than half of my life, but at different milestones — like my wedding, my first child being born, my son as well — it comes up again when you are looking around for some guidance or love, to share the moment. My daughter, Clara, is three now and she started saying, 'My nanna got that for me,' or 'In my dreams my nanna did this.' My husband's mother is called Grandma and she didn't have a nanna; I didn't know where this came from. So I showed her a picture of my mum and asked, 'Is this your nanna?' and she said, 'Yes.' Now she talks about her all the time — Nanna is not here because her body stopped working; she used to skip rope with her nanna; Nanna told her to swim between the flags. And now I tell Clara my own childhood stories about her nanna, and it's been wonderful to share my mum with her in this way.

LAUREN: Trees for Mum started off when Deena and I were talking about the motherless community. It was coming close to Mother's Day, so we said, 'Why don't we do something for Mother's Day?' Everywhere you looked there was advertising for Mother's Day; there were cards showing blonde kids running to blonde mothers with a present, and you just think, 'What about me?' I felt very excluded at that time of year. We came up with the idea that people could plant a tree in memory of their mums on Mother's Day and do something positive for her and give a purpose to the day. You would actually have something to go to on the day, so you wouldn't think that day was a void in your life when everyone else was out celebrating.

We have people whose mothers have died 40, 50 years ago who are still very much grieving, and then others whose loss has been in the last couple of weeks and they are so grateful to have something positive to do. So we see every stage of the grief process through Trees for Mum, and it just keeps growing and growing. We planned the first year without expecting anything to come out of it; we thought it was going to be a one-off. All of a sudden there were 150 people saying, 'Where are we going next year?' This year 8000 people participated across the country, and we've had interest from overseas. So it's snowballing to a point where we need some structure around it, so we don't turn into a snowball as well!

DEENA: We learned through experience when people asked, 'Where is my tree?' that some were getting attached to their particular tree. Most understand that all trees don't thrive and some do die, though we have had a few people get very upset. At some sites people write little messages on bamboo stakes and stick them next to their tree; we explain the stake won't be there forever, but they can come back and enjoy the growth of the whole area. Overall the feedback we get from those who participate is positive and very touching. Trees for Mum has been very rewarding for me — it's a great feeling to share this with the community.

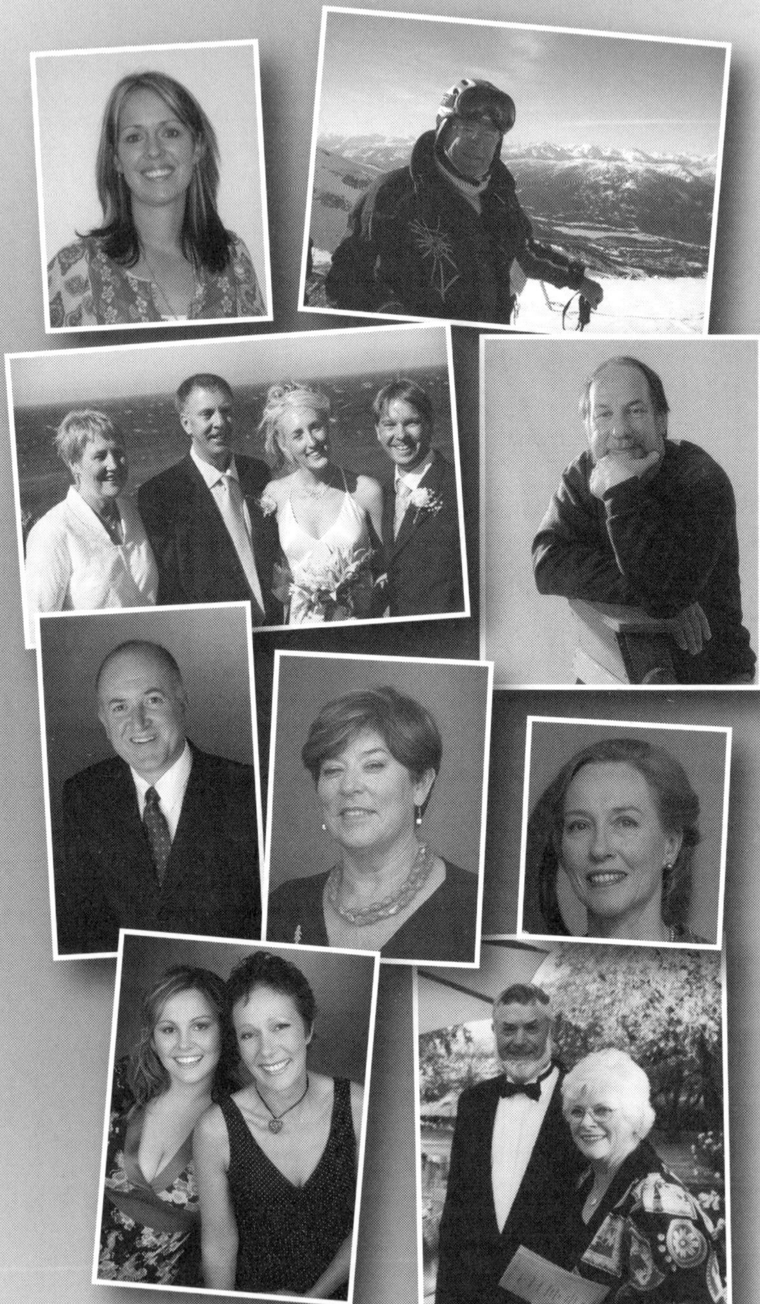

CHAPTER 5

The circle of compassion

> Suffering is but another name for the teaching of experience, which is the parent of instruction and the schoolmaster of life.
>
> **Horace (65 BC–8 BC)**

Generosity is a touchstone for many cancer survivors. They find that giving back is part of their healing process, and a way of ensuring that all that they've gone through hasn't been in vain. Many look for ways they can help others on their own 'cancer journey': some may establish cancer support groups or become a part of programs like the Cancer Council's Connect, which puts patients in touch with a volunteer with a similar cancer experience.

It's the 'cancer club' at work: a University of Newcastle study (funded by The Cancer Council NSW) showed that many cancer patients feel that the only people they could truly open up to were those who had gone through a comparable experience themselves. Those in the midst of diagnosis and treatment yearn to connect with those who have already walked that particular walk — and in this circle of compassion, the people doing the giving find that they, too, gain more than they imagined.

What starts as a connection becomes a life direction for some. Lyn Swinburne set up Breast Cancer Network Australia to assist other women finding their way through the 'battlefield' of breast cancer. Mohamed Khadra stepped away from life as a surgeon to set up a private university that would enable students in developing countries to study for an Australian degree. Tania Menzies used her expertise in establishing and running a successful nanny and babysitting service to set up a community nanny program for cancer patients. Lee Murphy is pursuing her passion for music, taking risks and stepping off her planned path so that she doesn't die wondering, 'What if?'

For each of them, cancer is not the end. It's a beginning.

Lyn Swinburne

What drives me is that basic concept about turning a negative into a positive. I think by nature we want to give back somehow. Most people I've met are incredibly generous; if you say to somebody, 'This is the help that I need,' then it is very rare for them to say to me, 'No, I can't do it.'

Lyn Swinburne was diagnosed with breast cancer in 1993 and underwent surgery, radiotherapy, chemotherapy and hormone therapy. She founded Breast Cancer Network Australia (BCNA) to ensure that women with breast cancer receive the best information, treatment, care and support. Now CEO of BCNA, Lyn is focused on making sure that women and families have a better experience after diagnosis than she did. 'That should be across the board in Australia, not just the people who can afford it, not just for people who live in the city, not just for people who can speak English or already have support,' she says. 'It is about setting a high standard of care and support and then making sure that is available to a whole lot of people.'

LYN SWINBURNE: It is quite easy to see positives when you come out the other side and you are well, but I get to meet a lot of women with advanced disease and many of those women can even see positives right through the incredible challenges they face, both physical and emotional. Not all the time — they have some very dark days. It is extraordinary, but somehow [cancer] reminds us about basic things that we sometimes forget when we are in the hurly-burly of life. We get caught up with stuff that doesn't matter; sometimes it is a chance to say, 'Stop.' All the little details are eroded away from you so you are taken back to your elements. Maybe sometimes in that clarity, you get to see things like you haven't seen them before.

It was very important for me to make positives in my life, because I found the experience of my breast cancer terrible. There weren't that many positives for me in the early days, to tell you the truth. I really struggled; I spent a lot of time hiding under the doona. I had two little kids, aged six and eight, and I was really worried that I wouldn't see them grow up. It was a very tough time. I also felt disempowered — a word that may be overdone a bit. Up until then in my life, if I met with an obstacle I had confidence in my own ability to get through it. Yet for the first time I felt that no matter what I did, it wouldn't matter. I had this strange thing growing in me and it was going to do what it was going to do, and whatever I did didn't really matter. That was incredibly disempowering, but little by little I thought, 'No, I can't let this take me over.' I'd had a great life and I wanted it back again; I wasn't prepared to say, 'That's the way it goes.' I needed to turn the crappy things that were happening to me into something that was going to be of value — mostly to me, to be honest. I wanted to do that so I could recapture my life, but then as I went on I was able to take a little step away and see what was happening to me and to other women. Little by little I realised that I had incredible advantages that not all women have: I had mates in the medical world who could say, 'Go to this doctor, go to this hospital, get a second opinion'; I had fantastic support from family and friends; neighbours with casseroles, people minding the kids; I had the ability to afford childcare on the days I felt like crap; we could get a babysitter in or go on a holiday; I was a confident, well-educated person — but it was excruciatingly difficult for me at that time. I started to think, 'For God's sake, if this is the gold standard of care I'm getting, what must it be like for others who don't have those advantages?' I used to wonder about [someone like] a single mother living in a high-rise flat in summer — how could she possibly manage? Or people who couldn't speak English very well, or people who didn't have family or support and were just shunted from pillar to post. I began thinking, 'If this is the best we can do, the worst must be unbearable,' and that became my personal motivation. I wanted it to be better for me but in trying to make it better for other people it also brought advantages for me, because I had a mission to take on.

If it hadn't been for having cancer, I wouldn't have done it all. Never in a million years. Mind you, I was always a person who did a lot of community things: I was president of the kindy, I was a primary school teacher and loved it. But it's really only the work that I've done since then that has revealed all sorts of things I had there sitting inside me: skills and talents that I'm sure would never have been unearthed had I not had this experience — like the confidence of public speaking. Somebody said to me the other day, 'You spoke at Telstra Stadium in front of 13,000 people and a TV audience of I don't know how many; that is extraordinary.' I never stopped to think about that because I was so caught up in the hurly-burly of it, and yet for some people, speaking in front of ten people is terrifying. I don't even think about that now; I enjoy it, I thrive on it. Most people I talk to who have experienced cancer do the opposite: they've had a busy life and then they say, 'Cancer has shown me I need to stop and I need to get rid of busyness.' But I'm the opposite; I feel driven.

Definitely my life now is very exciting and challenging as a result. I've had the opportunity to meet world leaders, I've carried the Olympic torch, I speak at overseas conferences, I've met lots of incredibly interesting people. It is an extraordinary life really, and it's because I had cancer. The other positive side is hearing from women who say, 'I got so well looked after, I had all these questions for the doctors but I got the answers.' All that is a source of extraordinary satisfaction to me because I feel I've played some sort of role in changing that system.

It takes a long time to change a system. Sometimes you despair and think it is never going to get better. [I did have a benchmark.] A person very close to me who helped me a lot when I was diagnosed with breast cancer — and she saw what I went through at close range, the difficulties I encountered, the lack of information and the lack of thought about how I was managing. She was then diagnosed herself with breast cancer something like 12 years after my experience. Now she's been through her own experience, and we agree the difference is extraordinary.

What drives me is that basic concept about turning a negative into a positive. I think by nature we want to give back somehow. Most people I've met are incredibly generous. If you say to somebody, 'This is the help that I need,' then it is very rare for them to say to me, 'No, I can't do it.' I am bowled over by the way people are generous —

and I don't just mean with money, but with their time. I talk to women in little country towns who have devoted their lives — they had breast cancer 25 years ago and they still run support groups and have a cup of tea together and they love that. It gives them back so much, to think they can help other people. It is that feeling that you are actually making the world a better place; it is a wonderful feeling to have somebody say, 'You've inspired me.'

Bad things can happen, and people can either respond by rising above it or being totally devastated. It is a very interesting thing about human nature: in life you see people choose to put a positive spin on something or choose to put a negative spin on it. I think often it is the way you are brought up: whether you are encouraged to look at a certain situation and make of it what you can. On the other hand, sometimes external stuff just makes it too hard. I've seen some courageous, tough, positive women who've been knocked down so many times, it is then too hard to get up that last time.

Sometimes we can help people deal with the external things. The lack of information, the feeling they are totally alone, the poor experience trying to communicate with the doctor — those are things we can do something about. We don't know what causes breast cancer, we can't stop it yet, so what we have to do is look after the people who are diagnosed and make it better for them. We can reduce those external pressures: the financial constraints, for instance. And we need to look after the women who have to travel huge distances for treatment, who have to come to the city for six weeks for radiotherapy — some of those women have never been to the city.

We often have huge expectations for ourselves. I would say to someone newly diagnosed, 'Take it one step at a time; just bite off as much information as you can chew; be gentle on yourself.' We hear stories of survival and positivity and we want to be in that place, but it can take a long time to get there. In an endeavour to get to that place, women often put a lot of pressure on themselves. I've heard women say, 'I've had my breast off and I'm standing here at the kitchen sink crying. I should be getting on with my life — why am I like this?' It's because they've had a huge assault on themselves — physically, emotionally — their whole life tree has been shaken. Sometimes you just have to be a bit gentle on yourself and say, 'That time will come,' but you have to wait for that time to come, to get to that headspace. For me it wasn't immediate — oh, God no. It took me two years to even realise that I felt better. Every single day I used to wake up and think, 'I've got cancer.' Then one day I suddenly thought, 'Oh, this is what it feels like to be right again.' You are assaulted from so many different directions; it is often the treatment that assaults you more than anything. You are facing big, big questions like, 'Am I going to survive?', 'What will happen to my children?', 'How will I tell my parents?', 'What will I do about work?', 'How am I going to get through the night with all this running around in my head?' Then comes, 'How do I understand the system, the words they use, the oncology stuff?' — it is so foreign — and there are all the clinical decisions you have to make. With breast cancer there are a lot of decisions: 'Will I try to save my breast? Is it better to go for big treatment and maximise my chance of survival? But what is that going to do to me in the long term?' It is a battlefield: your body is assaulted with the physical stuff, but also there is this incredible assault on who you thought you were; [now you are] this person who is no longer fearless. The system itself creates this faceless person and you wonder who on earth you are then.

It's not like that all the time; there are little bits and pieces of gorgeous moments in there — people telling you how important you are in their lives who would never have told you before. I've still got a box where I keep all the cards people sent to me when I was diagnosed; when I'm struggling or having a down time, I often just sit and open the box and read the cards. People have written things to me that are so precious; they would never have told me those things — they probably would have said them at my funeral. But people took the time to write those cards, so I like to say to people that when someone has been diagnosed or something happens that is a big challenge in their life, tell them how precious they are to you. Don't just send an SMS message — do that as well, but actually put it in writing that can be kept. Cancer is one of those things that gives you the opportunity to do those things we should all do.

I would love for cancer to be cured, but that is maybe not achievable — in our lifetime, at least. I think more likely there will be ways to better identify people at risk and to help them avoid the risks. My ultimate dream is that all people get the best treatment, care and support when they are diagnosed — so we can offer them the best chance of not only surviving, but surviving really well. So that their lives are more positive rather than less positive as a result of it. That would be my dream.

Mohamed Khadra

Life is so short, I just want to undo my belt and drink the whole lot, experience it all. That is my philosophy — whether that was a result of cancer or not, I don't know, but certainly cancer was a catalyst in making me more brave, to cut the rope that bound me to the mooring and make the boat go in different directions.

When he was faced with a diagnosis of thyroid cancer, Mohamed Khadra's mind went into overdrive. A professor of surgery, he had written papers on thyroid cancer for medical journals: 'I knew the numbers and statistics as well as anybody in Australia at the time.' After completing his treatment, Khadra left behind a successful career as a surgeon to pursue a new passion: he co-founded the Institute of Technology Australia (IOTA), a 'virtual university' with a social justice agenda,

offering an affordable Australian degree to students in developing countries through online learning.

MOHAMED KHADRA: The diagnosis of cancer forces you to evaluate whether the direction of your life is what you want it to be or whether you've been on a wave of life's forces, a leaf on a river. There is a difference between a life made and a life that has happened. The things I wanted to do were going to be later, after everything else — well, there may not be a later. So suddenly you think, 'What is it I want to fill each day with?'

The first thing I did was get out of the job I was doing, where I felt very little in the way of control. I was able to liberate myself from that and move north to Coffs Harbour. Then an opportunity I really wanted came up in England, and other activities occurred which I have been able to make use of because I was happy to cut the cord that bound me to my present.

Before my diagnosis I was much more childlike, much more ready to compromise myself to please others, whereas now I want to care for others but I also want to make sure my life is what I want it to be — 'To thine own self be true.'

I think [the change in me] was also partly me growing up. In the ten years between 37 and 47, you do a lot of growing up, just as you do between 16 and 26. That period in the 40s is a period where you need to re-evaluate, and if you don't re-evaluate then, often it's not done until the late 60s. Around the time of my cancer, a professor of anaesthetics at the hospital where I worked decided that after his retirement he was going to go to Vienna to study fine arts. His tickets were sitting on his mantelpiece, then the night before he was due to go he had a massive heart attack and died. It certainly affected a lot of people in the hospital. That added to the cancer experience for me — often there are different events that occur all at once, aligning one's life to a point where you say, 'I really have to change my life; this is not the direction I want to take.'

The journey is taken not only by you but those around you. I savour my children's lives more now: I got cancer when my youngest son was a year old and my eldest was about two, so they were very young at the time. I must say up until then I wasn't much of a father, but I've subsequently become a very involved father. I think your wife goes through it as well. It depends on what your relationship is like beforehand: ours was a very strong one, so it's almost like a team effort. That is an incredibly powerful life line that you have: you've got that support, you really want to make it through.

You soon find out your fair-weather friends and the people who will stick by you. In one fell swoop there were a substantial number of our friends — who we had thought were strong friends — who just disappeared, and then others very surprisingly came to the fore. So it does let you know who's on your side and who is not. It's not just people who have cancer: people who get divorced, or people who lose their jobs, or people who have any major event seem to report that the people around them are divided into two camps. There are people who avoid them like the plague, who just don't want to talk about those issues and if they do, it is very superficial; and then there are people who are really happy to cook a meal and bring it around and do very simple things which mean the world. I remember one particular event where my family were saying, 'Why does this happen to us?' that is, my illness had happened to them. It was quite obnoxious — they weren't going through it, I was. So that really ended my relationship with my family. I find it easier and easier to believe in reincarnation: I think the people who are old lives, old souls, are able to cope with cancer a lot better, whereas the vast majority seem to be naive, almost immature.

I did ask 'Why me?' a lot later, but not at the time. At the time it was very clinical, it was almost like a third party going through it. With my supervisor, the professor of surgery at Royal North Shore Hospital, where I was registrar at the time, I had written papers in the *Australian and New Zealand Journal of Surgery* on thyroid cancer, so it was almost like just adding up the statistics or seeing somebody else going through it. I organised my own treatment in a sense, because I knew what needed to happen. When the radiologist was passing the ultrasound probe around my neck, I knew what he was looking at and I realised [the cancer] was metastatic: it had gone into my neck, it had gone into my chest. All of that I realised on the first day, and I knew the numbers and statistics as well as anybody in Australia at the time.

After that initial period where I was organising everything, I suddenly realised this wasn't the way it should happen. I should be looked after, not look after myself. I said to my doctor, 'I just want to be an ordinary patient.'

Some people say it makes you a more compassionate or a better surgeon because you are able to feel what the patients are going through. I felt it made me a worse surgeon. You need to be able to have a dispassionate view of the body on that operating table, so every time you clamp an artery you are not lumbered with knowing what that responsibility is like, knowing what the family would feel like if this person passed away. Every time you sit across the desk from somebody, looking at their results, then announce to them their biopsy is positive — it became increasingly difficult for me to do my job objectively. It wasn't just an overnight thing; it took a number of years of me trying to do less and less surgery and more of everything else to realise I was actually trying to get away from it. Finally I just decided, this was the day. You know the old saying, 'When in doubt, cut it out'? It was easier to cut it out and have nothing to do with surgery than to prevail day by day in something that had lost its appeal to me and become much more painful than it should be.

I lived for surgery and there is an enormous part of me that misses it. I miss being in theatre, I miss operating, I miss all of that, but at some stage or other in my life I would have given it up. I can't be a surgeon till the day I die; the technical abilities do wane, so whether I gave it up at 65 or

45 — it was probably more sensible for me to give it up at 45, I suspect.

There are some people who see only one eventuality in their life and there are some of us who see multiple eventualities. My colleagues in other professions will change career every seven years; if you are in the corporate sector, you are constantly moving through different manifestations of yourself and different careers. You start off as a lawyer, then you might go into marketing, then maybe run a super fund. In surgery you start off as an 18-year-old doing medical school and at 65 you hang up your scalpel. In those ensuing 45 years you spend 15 training to become a surgeon and 30 being a surgeon, and then somebody taps you on the shoulder and says, 'Look, your results aren't as good as they used to be, maybe you should start thinking about giving it up.' So there were other parts of me that I had to explore, like considering being an educator or a businessman or maybe going off and doing law. Some people see that as a negative; they think, 'This person doesn't stick at anything; they haven't dedicated their whole life to doing one thing.' I see it as a positive: life is so short, I just want to undo my belt and drink the whole lot, experience it all. That is my philosophy — whether that was a result of cancer or not, I don't know, but certainly cancer was a catalyst in making me more brave, to cut the rope that bound me to the mooring and make the boat go in different directions.

I've always believed in an afterlife. I was brought up a very strict Muslim. I became far less religious when I got cancer than I was before — I started drinking the day I got cancer. I stopped praying when I got cancer, but I got much more spiritual. I became much more in tune with a sense of a life beyond this life, and much more open to the concept that people have multiple paths to tread to find their own spirituality. So the afterlife is not something that scares me. Death isn't something that scares me — I don't know why; I have never been scared of death. I'm scared of dying poorly, I don't want to linger in desperate pain or be a burden to those around me, but I am not afraid of the end result.

Karen Forster

I haven't let cancer define me, I've used it as an opportunity to grow … Fundamentally I am still the same person, I'm still the daughter, the sister, the mother that I was, but there are some habits that are no longer the same … I've done things that I've always wanted to do, changed my job, but I've also tried to do something positive with my life. I don't want to be there in a box and somebody saying, 'She had cancer and that was it.'

At the age of 41, Karen was diagnosed with invasive breast cancer. She underwent surgery and treatment over a 12-month period and has been cancer-free for eight years. She was also the primary carer for her husband, Danny, who died in 2007

from paranasal sinus cancer. After many years working in an educational environment, Karen now writes cancer policy and undertakes cancer-related research, and is a passionate advocate for cancer-related issues. She lives in Tasmania and has three adult children.

KAREN FORSTER: In a lot of ways I haven't let cancer define me, I've used it as an opportunity to grow and I think my children have as well. People say it changes your life, and that's definitely so for me: my life has changed quite dramatically. Fundamentally I am still the same person, I'm still the daughter, the sister, the mother that I was, but some habits have altered, and I know that applies to my children, too. We've tried to use it as a positive experience; we can learn from it and hopefully help other people as well along the way. I've done things that I've always wanted to do, like change my job, but I've also tried to do something positive with my life. I don't want to be there in a box with somebody saying, 'She had cancer, and that was it.'

I'm lucky to have had nine really good years and I know that is not always the case for other people with cancer. Many people are not as fortunate as me: they don't have family support, they don't have wonderful friends surrounding them with love and attention. They also don't have the education or the ability to seek out information or support, either; a lot of people need help to get that. The way I was brought up, part of what you do in life is help other people — through charity work, being involved in a service organisation or whatever. But now, as well as doing the things I've always done, I've brought in this part of my life and my experiences as well. I have three children who are in their 20s, and all of us are involved, whether it be raising funds, raising the profile of cancer, or public speaking. My middle child, who is a doctor, does quite a bit of public speaking about what it is like to have a mother [with cancer]. He was 16 when I was diagnosed, and that is a difficult time for a boy, but now he is trying to talk to people about what it's like and how families can help each other to come through these sorts of things.

When my children were tiny I worked at various things — as you do to be able to spend time with them and earn some money. When they were in primary school, I went back to work in administration, and then I worked at a school as a PR officer. It was during that time I was diagnosed with breast cancer. Schools really are communities in themselves, and that community of people was extremely supportive and wonderful to me and helped me through by offering flexible working hours et cetera. Facing your own mortality, you ask, 'What have I done with my life?' and one of the things I knew I hadn't done was fulfilled my potential for study. In some ways that was a disappointment to my parents, because I had been accepted into university when I left school but chose to take a job instead. I thought, 'Well, right now that is what I'm going to do for myself.' Exactly 12 months after my breast cancer diagnosis I enrolled in uni; still being a mother and being a wife, I was working 25 hours a week and doing part-time study. I continued with that until I took long service leave and I finished my degree full time. Towards the end of my course, a job opportunity arose where I am working now, as a community educator for breast screening. My father was alive at the time and he said to me, 'That job is made for you; you should apply for that.' Dad was extremely excited and he felt very positive about it. Then he died very suddenly; the interview for the job was on the day of his funeral. I wondered, 'Can I do this?' — and I did. Subsequently I got the job and knew that it was meant to be.

Following my breast cancer diagnosis I had become involved in breast cancer advocacy work through Breast Cancer Network Australia, so I had gained an incredible breadth of knowledge. My job was going out into the community convincing women to be 'breast aware' and have mammograms. I didn't use my own experience as leverage but there were times when I did share that, when it was appropriate to discuss that experience. [When I became a full-time community educator] I needed to know more about the health sector so I commenced some postgraduate studies in health promotion, which I completed this year, finally — I had to leave it for a little while when my husband was sick. Late last year I moved into policy development and policy writing — not just for breast cancer but for all cancers. Now I am involved in a lot of exciting cancer-related projects; we have some groundbreaking things happening in the reorganisation of the health system here in Tasmania. I've been involved in setting up a cancer advocacy network in the State, so now I'm called upon to be the voice of people with cancer here in Tasmania, on government-related committees and forums. I could not have imagined ever being asked to speak about these sorts of things before. Three years ago I was doing something I'd done for quite a long time and never imagined that anything would be any different.

You can wallow in your own misery and say, 'Why did this happen to us?', and there are moments when you do that. But then you look at the other side and say, 'What is the reason that it did happen? What can we learn? What can we take from that?' Instead of saying, 'Why me?' say, 'Well, it is me, it is us; what can we do to turn it into a positive experience?' That's a new fundamental our family adopted. That was something my husband taught the teachers, the other staff and the principal at the school where he worked; he also taught the students about how to live with something like that in a positive way — he taught teenage boys a lot about dying.

Sally Crossing

Nobody wants to know about cancer if they can help it. If I hadn't been diagnosed with cancer, I would not have even considered trying to improve the cancer journey … But the combination of giving back and being able to make things change for the better is very heady stuff.

Utterly pragmatic and business-like, Sally Crossing's response to being diagnosed and treated for breast cancer in 1995 and 2004 was to use her expertise in government policy-making to benefit the 'breast cancer community'. She founded the Breast Cancer Action Group NSW (Australia) in 1997 and is Chair of Cancer Voices NSW. In 2005 she was appointed a Member of the Order of Australia (AM) for her services to the community.

SALLY CROSSING: When I was first diagnosed in 1995 with early-stage breast cancer, I was busy working as a policy director of a State government department. I had a full-time job, a husband, two teenage children, a Sydney house, a farm and a dog — I was busy being one of those women who wanted to do it all and have a full and satisfying life. So a diagnosis of breast cancer was a big shock. The rug is pulled from under your feet — you think you are standing very firmly, you have created this life and then suddenly it is all quite likely to be a house of cards and collapse.

I had a bad experience with my first diagnosis because my GP referred me to a general surgeon who didn't do anything for some time, and then finally did something which turned out to be inadequate. That disturbed me quite a lot, although I didn't know any better then. You never really thought you had to know what was wrong with you and needed to be involved in making informed decisions; this is something you learn later on. Luckily I then fell into the hands of a specialist breast surgeon and had proper treatment, although in hindsight things were missed even then.

When I knew I wasn't going to die there was a big sigh of relief and everything went back to normal. I turned 50 about six months after all the treatment; I'd continued working throughout it. After a while I began to think about the things that had happened to me. I wrote an article, a reflective piece about what had happened, and gave it to the National Breast Cancer Centre. They printed it in one of their publications and invited me to go to Melbourne to do a course on consumer advocacy and science training. I met a couple of compelling women down there: Sue Lockwood [Chair of the Breast Cancer Action Group Victoria], who subsequently became very sick with advanced breast cancer, and Lyn Swinburne, who now runs the Breast Cancer Network Australia. We all remember walking around a park and saying there is nothing happening in New South Wales. They both said, 'You ought to go and do it because you have the skills and the passion.' So I said, 'Well, I'll think about it if you will undertake to help and support me,' because they had been doing breast cancer advocacy work for three years.

I went back to New South Wales and started up the Breast Cancer Action Group NSW. There was an article in the *Sydney Morning Herald* in October 1997, announcing our start-up, with a big photo of the three of us in the Art Gallery. The photographer had taken us around all these beautiful artworks of bare breasts and we finally settled on a bronze torso, with two obviously perfect breasts — between us we had two and a quarter! When we met just this year

[2008] to celebrate our first decade of making a difference for women with breast cancer, we only had one between us ... That was the beginning of the Breast Cancer Action Group in New South Wales.

After a while I decided to retire early from my job, not just because of the breast cancer experience, but also I could see the advocacy area was picking up steam and that real differences could be made. I was then able to spend more time on the group. One of the first major projects was [publishing] the *Directory of Breast Cancer Treatment and Services in New South Wales*, which came immediately out of my experience — which I found to be a common one — that GPs just didn't know where to refer people for best outcomes. It doesn't only happen in breast cancer, it happens in all cancers. So we have developed this template, which is now electronic, national, regularly updated, and the first of its kind in the world.

There is so much I've learned from the breast cancer experience. It means I've been able to give back, and my country has honoured me for doing so — I have been awarded an AM. The experience has changed my life. Although I was using similar skills inside a State government department, it was frustrating because it took ages for anything to happen. Because we operate outside the system, we find ourselves having a broader view than anybody else and freedom to express it where it matters. I was sitting at a Cancer Institute NSW meeting yesterday asking the sort of high-level questions which the others didn't immediately see, and they all came out saying, 'Yes, that's what we need.' So it is very exciting, stimulating and satisfying. Expanding the breast cancer work to cancer in general was a logical next step — so many of the needs are the same. Over the last ten years I hope, and I think, I've made a difference.

Nobody wants to know about cancer if they can help it. If I hadn't been diagnosed with cancer, I would not have even considered trying to improve the cancer journey; I wasn't interested in health. When you are in the throes of your career, your kids and your life, you can't commit your time to something like this. People occasionally say, 'You middle-aged educated women, how can you be speaking for all these women?' Well, someone's got to do it, someone who is able to do it, and if it's not done, all those others miss out on the benefits. We are all volunteers; nobody funds us (other than private donors), and we want to remain entirely independent. One of the big challenges is finding other keen people, finding out what they can do and working with their skills and interests.

One of the many positives is it makes you feel good that you are doing something worthwhile, and it is nice to be recognised as having done so. To be honest, I guess self-esteem is part of it, too.

It is a community of shared experiences. We just had a breast cancer information and advocacy forum for 150 women at Sydney University. There was a feeling of coming together with people you wouldn't otherwise get to know, all with a set of experiences in common. It is a bit like an exclusive club — not one you would apply for! We all know we look at life differently now.

When I was diagnosed with advanced breast cancer in 2004, it was another huge shock — and a huge mortality check for me. When you've got early-stage cancer, your chances of survival are pretty good these days. Being diagnosed with advanced disease is different. I said, 'What is the average survival period?' and my specialist said, 'Four years'. Four years — that really hits home. I decided to be one of those on the long statistical tail beyond four years. I go to a support group for people with advanced breast cancer at Royal North Shore Hospital. A lot of them are much further down the track than I am, and it is very interesting listening to them — some of them are coping, some aren't; some live with it as a chronic condition; one ended her own life; but there is still a strong bond between us.

A couple of people have also said to me that I have become a professional consumer advocate: very into the issues, committees, the advocacy side of things — perhaps not in touch enough with real people. I suppose when you've been doing it for a long time, you do tend to think in bigger-picture, policy-type terms — at the level where change-making decisions are made. On the other hand, we as a group (both BCAG NSW and Cancer Voices NSW) absolutely recognise that to be credible, you have to be in touch with the grass roots and real people. And getting a diagnosis and losing a breast and half your liver does ground you personally.

I get such a buzz doing something I know I can do well and that actually has results. I retired from paid work at 51; I am now 61, and it is good to feel engaged. The family sometimes suffers because I disappear: I'm busy or not in contact or speaking at conferences or travelling. I have a very supportive husband. We had a discussion just recently; he's 64 and he said, 'I can't retire until you do,' because I'd still be whizzing about on cancer consumer advocacy and he'd be wanting to do things with me. We'll have to work that one out …

I think I have personally grown as a result of my cancer experience. The two diagnoses had slightly different impacts; the second one really focused me on mortality and stepping back and having another look at life, because it could be considerably shortened. One of my daughters was giving me a lecture about my care of my 88-year-old mother and she said, 'Mum, you must spend more time with her and make sure she doesn't feel you're doing it out of duty.' And then she said, 'You wouldn't want me to feel that when you're old,' and I said, 'But you are lucky — I won't be so old.' I'll shuffle off well and truly before 88 and I don't mind that.

I went through the whole thing about facing death and realised that there isn't a sting for the person who dies, the sting is for the ones who wish you hadn't. For me, it is the way of dying that disturbs me; I would like to have control over that. I will want to know exactly what my prognosis is, what my treatment and palliation options are, and get more than one opinion on them. I also want to die the way I want to die, so I've done a bit of research on that. A lot of people do because they resent having to hand themselves over, when they are very sick and in pain, to the control of other people, who may or may not respect their dignity and wishes.

Dying is not much on my mind; I've been through that, I've thought it through, I am happy with that. It is no good fretting about it.

Lisa Humphries

I am just doing whatever I can to make sure my experience isn't wasted — I feel I've been given this gift of insight into people living every day with cancer. It is to honour my mother as well … I think I inherited her spirit, which I saw put to the ultimate test when she had to live with cancer for six years and never complained. I feel like I am a completely different person because of it, a better person.

When she was in her 20s, Lisa was the primary carer for her mother, who died of breast cancer in 2000. Lisa cared for her mother full-time for three years and part-time for another three years. Out of that experience, Lisa has found a passion to share her experience and to help others on a similar journey. She is familiar with the darker side of caring, too, having come through years of depression and anxiety (a common outcome for people caring for those with cancer).

LISA HUMPHRIES: My mum survived a lot longer than the doctors predicted; her original prognosis was not good, yet she lived for six years. I never expected that I would be caring for her for that long; it just went on and became such a big part of my life.

I didn't know a lot about cancer prior to my mum being diagnosed; until it touches you, it is not something you choose to learn about. Just by spending so much time in hospital, I started to see all these people caring for people with cancer and this connection we all had; people were always looking out for each other. When you are [at someone's side] in intensive care, when you are in the oncology ward, strangers are connected by this horrible disease, and that is when I started to see how powerful our spirit becomes when we are faced with horrible things like cancer. I started to develop more of that in myself and I saw it in my mother. She lived with this incredibly painful cancer that spread through all her bones. She was having pins put in her limbs and she never complained, she never got upset — not in front of me, anyway. I saw this amazing spirit; she wanted her kids to see her deal with this; she never let it show she was in pain. I saw this spirit in her and other people that were living with this thing; it illuminated me in so many ways as well as saddened me.

It was not that I was a selfish person before, it was just that I was existing in my own world and not looking outside my existence. Once I saw all these people living with cancer and became one of this group of people who cared or who lived with someone with cancer, I slowly became more and more inspired to move into that field in my career.

A year after Mum passed away, I stood up at my desk in my corporate job and quit on the spot, then I went to try to start my own charity. I lost all my savings in the process. I was determined I was going to change the world and eventually I realised it was going to be a little bit difficult to do that on my own. I had no experience in the charity sector, so I went to work for a charity. That was about four years ago now, and I slowly worked my way up into managing a patient support program. Along the way I've done a lot of volunteer work as well: I've volunteered in hospitals with patients, I've volunteered for events and raised money, I joined Carers NSW and became a camp leader with them. Right now is a really pivotal time for me. Today is my last day working in fundraising; as of Monday I start working on a patient support program here at the Cancer Council. Seven years ago that was my dream. It is such an amazing feeling to know my life has led me to this point.

I am just doing whatever I can to make sure my experience isn't wasted — I feel I've been given this gift of insight into people living every day with cancer. It is to honour my mother as well. Her life was so short; she created these two amazing people in her children, and I feel proud to be able to share that with people. I think I inherited her spirit, which I saw put to the ultimate test when she had to live with cancer for six years and never complained. I feel like I am a completely different person because of it, a better person.

[The experience of nursing my mother has] changed a lot of my relationships and I've lost a lot of friends — not lost, but I've chosen to remove myself from people's lives. My values have changed, and it sometimes makes it hard to communicate with other people. I would never wish anything like I've been through on anyone, but I also see people who have been through something like [caring for a loved one with cancer] have a completely different outlook on life and I relate a lot better to those people. I get very frustrated when I see my friends complaining about something that doesn't matter in the big scheme of things. They would get along better with the old Lisa because she would be complaining about the same type of things. I don't get stressed in my car any more; I used to be this crazy 21-year-old who needed to get somewhere and that was all that mattered. Now if someone is driving really slowly in front of me I don't get angry with them; I think, 'They might be on their way to the hospital, or someone might have just died, or someone might be sick.' I just have this whole new range of thoughts that go through my head and they are all positive thoughts, so I'm grateful for that.

I feel things more intensely; I am more aware of my senses and my feelings. When I feel happy, it is a greater depth of happiness because I appreciate the fact that I am happy and I'm healthy. In a sense, it is about the simple things and being able to take pleasure in those, because I saw how quickly it can be taken away. I am here, I am breathing, I am healthy, I don't have to go to hospital. I just saw another side to life that people live with every day and I don't have to live with. Although I miss my mum and I will be grieving for a very long time, on the other hand I still feel very alive.

At the same time, I have a big fear of death now and a very intense awareness of my own mortality. Before I saw cancer first hand, I thought I was immortal, which a lot of people do when they are young. Until you see what something like cancer can do to someone so young, you don't think about it.

I've learned so much from my mother about how to be a good person — and how to be a good friend: she had so many great friends. I want to leave a bit of her with everyone I meet, and that comes out in the way I treat people: in my work, with my colleagues — just to be a person people can come to if they need someone to talk to, the person who will always listen. I also think I have a lot of capacity to love now and to give myself to people. I can't wait to have my own children and to be the type of mother she was to me, so that is quite exciting as well — to leave some of those traits in my own children.

I feel like every day I am living my mother's personality and her spirit and what she has taught me. That has changed me as well; when I make decisions or do things or speak to people, I feel like she is an influence on those things all the time. I learned a lot in seeing her life up until she was sick and while she was sick — you will never see a more gracious, tolerant, giving person. So she is with me all the time.

Jeff Winter

> *I got invited to go to a men's health forum to talk about cancer. I spoke of my first diagnosis. Devastating. I spoke of my second diagnosis. Even more devastating. I spoke of my concern for my family, our financial status turned upside down … When I finished there was not a sound. Not a movement. Not a question. The other speakers all came across and gave me a tight embrace. The audience stood and I remember the applause. Good feeling? You bet! It just felt good to be alive. The phone calls and questions started and have never stopped. To this day I have never turned down an invitation to speak and perhaps to pass on hope through personal experience. I'm still here. I plan to stay for a while.*

If you want to know the good and the bad that can come out of cancer, ask Jeff Winter. He has been there, and he doesn't pull any punches about the ups and the downs. In 2000, Jeff had just been given the all-clear for a cardio condition when his doctor noticed a suspicious mole on his back. It was found to be an aggressive melanoma, requiring immediate surgery. Five years later a routine chest X-ray revealed a tumour in his lung which turned out to be lung cancer. Another operation and painful rehabilitation followed. In the dark and often lonely days that followed, Jeff threw himself into fundraising, including volunteering on the Relay For Life Committee in Inverell. Relay For Life is a series of 24-hour fundraising events organised locally by volunteers in towns and suburbs across Australia. His committee raised $90,000 — an incredible amount from a town of 10,000 people.

JEFF WINTER: I had one cancer in 2000 and one in 2005. The first one, I was so blasé, I thought it did not matter. I was probably trying to cover it up; a bloke like me had everything going for him — a good life, a good family unit, good food and plenty of red [wine]. A lot of people get cancer once in their life, and I thought, 'Okay, that's mine.' I had plastic surgery on the damn thing, but I was just stupid; I thought I'd had my little brush now and it wouldn't come again. I was criticised for taking it so lightly. But with the second one, that is when it started to sink in. I knew I was in big trouble.

I think [my wife] Ann-Marie and I both handled it very badly. It happened so fast: on the Wednesday before Easter I was taken to John Hunter Hospital, and they sent me back home on Easter Sunday while they decided what to do. I got a call on Easter Monday to say, 'Get your bum in, we are operating tomorrow morning.' At that stage the kids were 15 and nine. Anthony, the 15-year-old, was in complete denial; he couldn't even say the word cancer, he would never come to hospital. Matthew, he's the youngest bloke, he decided he wanted to come down to Newcastle, to John Hunter. He stayed through every procedure, he wanted to know everything that was going on — 'What are you doing that to Dad for?', 'What's that in his arm?' After a week and a half he turned around and said, 'Mum, Dad's in good hands, I can go home now.'

I was there for about three-and-a-half weeks. When I came back home I had a choice of sitting in a corner and feeling sorry for myself or getting on with life. We'd made an advanced care plan at that stage as we thought I might not make it through to Christmas. One of the things I used to hate was when people would say, 'Think positively.' Think positively about what? I've got cancer! The other thing that used to really upset me was, 'I know how you feel.' You feel like saying, 'You don't know how I feel; you wouldn't have a clue.'

I was working for the Education Department in behaviour and welfare, trying to get 12-year-olds out of suspension and back into school, which I loved. Of course I had to give that up. In Coles, people would walk up the next aisle so they didn't have to talk to you. All of a sudden, the phone calls and invitations to barbecues stopped.

Matthew came home one night and said, 'They had show-and-tell at school but I didn't show, all I did was told.' He got up and told all the kids at school his dad had cancer, and we had to do something to beat it. It absolutely pulled the rug out from under us. I was not in remission, I was only home for a couple of months, and I decided I had to do something. I went to volunteer at a large retirement village with 200-odd people, one of the biggest employers in town. I started doing leisure activities for the old people, then I got invited to go to a men's health forum to talk about cancer — and I just ran from it completely. Ann-Marie had a very good go at me about feeling sorry for myself, so what I did was I went to the men's forum. I wrote a speech, and when it was my turn to get up in front of the lectern I forgot all about my speech; I just went from the heart and let it all pour out. Ninety-nine per cent of the people at that forum were local people from our small town, and that was my first coming out. Two years down the track it has absolutely snowballed. For the last 15 months I've been talking to men's groups — I just speak about it all, the good and bad.

I was hesitant as I had never made public my two cancer conditions — melanoma and lung cancer. I was not in remission at this stage. The other speakers were a health professional from Diabetes Australia, a pharmacist with a strong interest in prostate cancer and the CEO of a large retirement village. I felt in good company.

Being very nervous, I wrote and rehearsed a speech along the lines of what I thought they wanted to hear: don't smoke, don't drink, don't stay out in the sun, watch your diet, be nice to your neighbours and don't beat your wife and kids! I was last cab off the rank, and I patiently listened to the other keynote speakers. It was then that I realised that I was off with the fairies if I thought that this group would swallow my goody-goody words of wisdom. I remember I was becoming very emotional and I doubted if I could go through with this. I was worried that I was going to make a real goose of myself, in front of a lot of people who I knew. And more importantly, that I would embarrass my wife and two young boys — we live in a small town where everybody knows everybody.

But as I started to speak, the past came back to me. I spoke about long days on the beach at Surfers Paradise as teenagers, when the big thing was to get as brown as we could. I spoke of a marriage breakdown and my subsequent 'run and hide' in the coalfields of central Queensland. The lonely life of being in a camp of a thousand blokes where all you did was to raise the right hand — knowing that your alcohol levels were hitting alarm rates, but who cared? But all these things came back and haunted me. I spoke of my first diagnosis. Devastating. I spoke of my second diagnosis. Even more devastating. I spoke of my concern for my family, our financial status turned upside down.

Emotions ran high. I spoke of personal hardships, family relationships, how I had to give up my employment to claim superannuation. I spoke of being told of a second cancer. I spoke of being told of two other 'dormant cancers'. I could have gone on and on but I stopped on a positive note: the feeling of 'still being here' and getting on with my life. And hope!

When I finished there was not a sound. Not a movement. Not a question. The other speakers all came across and gave me a tight embrace. The audience stood and I remember the applause. Good feeling? You bet! It just felt good to be alive.

The phone calls and questions started and have never stopped. To this day I have never turned down an invitation to speak and perhaps to pass on hope through personal experience. I'm still here. I plan to stay for a while.

Anthony was still in denial; we had to pull him out of school in Year 10. His attitude went pear-shaped: his attitude towards us was absolutely shocking, his school work went down. We got him counselling, but that didn't work so we let him take his own pace. He is slowly coming around; he is 17 now. But the little bloke has been the light in my life. He wants to know what's going on — that's his way of coping. Anthony, on the other hand, he's always been a bit of a loner but when it came to this he just completely alienated himself from us, he wouldn't talk to us. Up to this day he has never said that word. One of the psychologists said, 'He has to go and say "cancer".'

Sure, there are some days I feel sorry for myself and I try not to think about it. I've had one lung taken out – that's why I'm puffing — and the other one has three nodes. There are two tumours, they are only small, stuck in the top lobe and while they are not doing anything, they don't really call it remission, but I have reached two years after the event.

Since this happened, I have done a lot of work for the Cancer Council and with a group called Cancer Connect. People with the same condition are matched up, and we talk about emotions, procedures, medication. When I get calls for that, it does affect me; I do get a bit withdrawn and I do have mood changes. My wife will tell you … but the Cancer Council is a great thing. I'm also involved in the Relay For Life event here. The relay is led out by survivors who are at different stages — again it is a 'coming out of the closet' thing. I recruited as many survivors as I could; I thought if I could get 50 survivors from a town like Inverell, that would be great. We had 274. It was just so brilliant — people like me who hadn't even talked about it were coming out and saying, 'I've had cancer.' That was a big buzz, that's for sure.

I think you go through stages. You go through the 'Why me? What have I done to deserve this?' For me in particular, 'Why have I got two goes at it?' Then you've got to get over it. There are big downsides to it, of course; at the moment there are more ups, but there are bad days. In the early stages, I felt sorry for myself. I hit the red, then I tried meditation. Now when I feel like it I say a little meditation or a prayer. Through it all our marriage has come a little bit unstuck. To this day it's not 100 per cent, but we are working on it.

Cancer runs in the family, which is really unfortunate. I feel for the kids and Ann-Marie; I give them more hugs and kisses now.

Colleen McKay

I guess I wanted to do something to make my mum and dad proud. My dad was diagnosed [with cancer] a month after my sister was diagnosed, and losing him has probably been the biggest thing I've ever dealt with. When he was dying, he said, 'Colleen, your life is about getting breast cancer out there.'

Some families seem to get hit by cancer from every direction. Colleen McKay's mother died of cancer when Colleen was 13 years old. In 1999 Colleen's sister was diagnosed with breast cancer when she was pregnant; after chemo and having a breast removed she is now healthy. Their father was found to have bowel cancer the month after her sister was diagnosed, and he passed away in 2006. Six weeks before that, his brother lost his battle with bowel cancer as well. Genetic testing showed that Colleen and her other two sisters and brother have the gene. Two weeks after receiving the test results, Colleen was diagnosed with breast cancer; she was breastfeeding her second daughter at the time. Colleen has since had chemo and a breast removed; she discovered she was pregnant with her third daughter, Polly, just after her final round of chemo. In September last year, Colleen had the other breast removed and both breasts reconstructed. After all of that, 'I had to do something just to see if I could get on top of things,' Colleen says.

Colleen McKay: Cancer has led me to running a young woman's support group in Ballarat. I am involved with Breast Cancer Network Australia [BCNA], which has led me to some wonderful places. I had the honour of tossing the coin for the beginning of the game at the 2007 Sydney Field of Women. [Before the Sydney Swans v St Kilda match, 13,000 women dressed in bright pink ponchos and 100 men in blue stood in formation in a statement of support for Australians affected by breast cancer.] I love the social life of it all; I've been to Sydney with BCNA, I did the *9am* TV show with David and Kim — [these are some of the] little things I love doing.

I attended the Melbourne Field of Women in 2005 too, and I have never experienced anything like it. That night, I thought so much of Mum and wished she had been there to share it with us. My brother and sister both were standing on the ground with me. It was very emotional, but it's an amazing feeling knowing that there are so many others feeling the same.

Because of our strong family history of cancer, it has always been in my life. I don't think until you've experienced it yourself you could go out and do what I am doing. I think I was diagnosed for a reason. I guess I wanted to do something to make my mum and dad proud. My dad was diagnosed a month after my sister was diagnosed, and losing him has probably been the biggest thing I've ever dealt with. When he was dying, he said, 'Colleen, your life is about getting breast cancer out there; you are the right person to advertise for it.' My dad was proud of me no matter what I do, but I think you just want to make them happy.

My daughter Tess was five, and Demi was a baby when I was diagnosed, so having another baby, having a hysterectomy, having both breasts off — there was just too much I had to deal with at once, and then losing my dad was like the last straw. I had to do something just to see if I could get on top of things. People say, 'Gosh, you dealt with breast cancer so well,' but people never saw the dark side, I'd never ever let anyone see it. The fear of dying was my main worry but I never let on about that to anyone else. [My husband] Dean was always so positive, telling me how beautiful I was with one breast, or no breast, it never ever worried him. He'd say, 'Col, it doesn't change what you are.' It would make you feel really good, but every morning you'd walk in [the bathroom] and in the mirror you'd see [your scarred chest]. It was a pretty hard thing to deal with; it is a womanly thing to have breasts.

I wanted to keep it together for Dean; I didn't want to let Dean see me fall in a heap. I just wanted to prove to my family that I was so strong. I've always been the strong one. I'm the baby out of five. I've always been the outspoken one, always organised everything and I just didn't want to fail. My life has been a challenge, always. My mum died 22 years ago at the end of this month; I was 13. Growing up with your father and five kids in the house, with no mother — it's always been challenging.

I am a very different person now, a better person, more open. I take life day to day; nothing worries me as much any more. It has made me a stronger person, it has made me meet people, it has made me have goals in life, which I've never really had before. I'm a qualified hairdresser. I owned a salon and sold that after I had my first baby, but now my goal is to put the awareness of breast cancer out there.

Geoff Whitelaw

Life doesn't end with prostate surgery; in fact it can give you a new lease of life … I encourage men to talk about the sexual side of things and what the possible side effects could mean for them. Some men say, 'It doesn't worry me,' but of course it does.

After undergoing radical prostate surgery in 1993 at the age of 53, Geoff Whitelaw found it difficult to know where to turn for information: back then, there simply wasn't much available. Although the surgery had eliminated the malignancy, he was both incontinent and impotent. Once he learned how to get on with life, he was determined to pass on his new knowledge to other men grappling with the same issues.

GEOFF WHITELAW: It took me three or four months to get my act together [after the surgery]. I remember there was a jazz festival on and I just decided I had to go. I went with a leg bag attached and I actually ended up getting up and dancing. I can remember that being a big turning point.

Psychologically I was through the emotional side in 12 months, but it was quite a change. I was a single guy and I'd had many relationships; to be suddenly hit with this situation was a bit of a problem.

Being an accomplished dancer gave me the confidence to be able to approach women. I could relate through dance. If I hadn't had that skill, if I'd met someone at a bar I don't think I'd be that confident to ask them home. The big process was getting over that question of what was going to happen to new relationships and how to get past that first theoretical hurdle — it is a theoretical hurdle but a real hurdle.

I'd certainly prefer things to be different — but I have a pretty good life. I don't think I've lost a female partner because of the problems I suffer from. I am fairly sure there have been some I haven't started to have a relationship with because people have said, 'He's impotent,' or 'He's incontinent.' I'm sure some guys have used the impotence thing against me, but to the best of my knowledge, the ladies I've been out with have not missed out too much.

[When I was diagnosed] I was an industrial chemist and I had sold my business to another company 12 months previously, but I was still operating a one-man business within their confines. I was going out to see electroplaters and talking to them; theoretically I was meant to be selling and marketing, but I found I was talking more to my customers about prostate cancer than electroplating technology. At that stage there was very little information available; I'd gone to the library and I'd picked up a few leaflets, but within that 12-month period it suddenly started to be noticed and mentioned on the radio and elsewhere. I was doing my own little bit on the side but about four years after that, a friend of mine at the Cancer Council decided to set up a prostate support group. I was part of that and have been the entire time it's been going.

The Cancer Help Line has a number of us who are there to offer support to people with similar situations. Tomorrow I'm going in to give a half-hour talk to a new group being trained on what it is like for me to offer that support. I also wrote a little piece on sex after radical prostatectomy, and it was picked up by the Cancer Council; I then gave a talk to prostate care nurses, and my three-page piece is still part of their training program. So I consider myself to be one of the people who are good at talking to others about the positive side and [reassuring them] that there is life after radical prostatectomy. I can say from experience that life doesn't end with prostate surgery; in fact it can give you a new lease of life.

I am quite sure the people I talk to on the phone do benefit. The girls [who call in: they may be cancer sufferers or friends or partners] seem to develop a relationship that keeps going, but for the guys, it is usually only two phone conversations: they get the information, and when you ring back they say, 'Oh yeah, I think I'm fine.' I encourage men to talk about the sexual side of things and what the possible side effects could mean for them. Some men say, 'It doesn't worry me,' but of course it does.

I'm lucky: I haven't had any PSA readings for over ten years. [PSA tests are used to screen for cancer of the prostate and to monitor treatment of the disease.] Pathology tests following my surgery showed that the cancer had just progressed into the seminal tract, so if I hadn't opted to have the operation as soon as possible, I may not have been alive and so fit and well today. However, I made the decision for the wrong reason. In truth I have given myself a bit of a hard time on whether I should have gone flat out and had the operation immediately or done a little more investigation. Part of that decision-making process was that I was working for this company and I wanted to have the surgery during the Christmas holidays. I pushed myself to get up earlier than I should: some clients were in trouble and I got in the car and went down there without urinary control. [I ended up having an accident and] it all went down my front, which was a bit embarrassing. I put the job ahead of my health, which I've done a couple of other times in my life. I would hope that I wouldn't do the same thing again.

Pauline Welch

> *I have learned so much in all the different things I've done since [having cancer], that I probably am different from what I was before ... I do feel a lot more confident, game to try different challenges.*

Five years after her diagnosis and treatment for breast cancer in 1992, Pauline Welch and her husband left behind their old life in Melbourne to run a bed and breakfast in the spectacular Grampians region, two-and-a-half hours northwest of Melbourne.

PAULINE WELCH: Cancer made my husband and me look at our life in Melbourne, think about what we were going to do, and get out of the rat race. We looked all over Victoria for the right spot. Once we realised this is what we wanted to do, we had so many weekends away looking at different areas, and we discovered the Grampians, which is such a beautiful, clean, peaceful spot. There were very few traditional B&Bs in the Grampians area, so we bought something that was really different. It was an octagonal house which we'd always looked at but never thought we'd have the chance to buy; it was just built as a family home, so we did some alterations and opened it as a B&B.

If it hadn't been for cancer, I think we would possibly still be living in Melbourne. My husband is a builder and he'd be hating the traffic, working all over Melbourne. At the time I was diagnosed, I had recently started a career as a Tupperware demonstrator. I don't do things by halves; three months into it, I was starting to think about becoming a manager. Then I was diagnosed, so all of that went out the window for about 12 months. I'm not quite sure what I'd be doing, but I'd probably be working there and hating it.

We've got a lot busier and bigger than we ever expected — as I said, we don't do things by halves; if you are going to do something you do it properly. After all the registrations and marketing and advertising, we got star rated: we are 4.5-star — I don't know if that means a lot to a lot of people, but it is a high standard. The area is absolutely beautiful; we are only ten minutes out of Halls Gap, in a beautiful place called Pomonal, and we are surrounded by about 4 acres of land and gardens. If it all gets too much, you go for a wander. And we just meet so many people from all over the world.

When I was diagnosed, the only person I had ever known who had breast cancer was my mother-in-law, who was deceased by then, so I didn't have anyone to ask all those funny little questions. My surgeon's nurse said, 'When you are symptom-free for a certain amount of time, you can go and do some training to help other people going through breast cancer.' So I did the training with what was then the Breast Cancer Support Service. It is now part of Cancer Connect, which has volunteers from all different cancers who speak to people going through the same thing. I've been doing that for over ten years now. It wasn't until the last five years that I realised that I had never been given the opportunity to talk to a support person myself. It didn't even occur to me to ask; whether they thought I didn't need it, I'm not quite sure. But it has been invaluable, both I think to the people I talk to and also to me. I like trying to help people through. When I'm on the phone to these ladies, quite often we both have a cry; I feel for them, I know what they are going through.

A lot of the literature now says, 'Let your friends look after you and do things.' One big thing I remember is that some friends used to call in and I'd be feeling really lousy, especially after chemo, but they'd be sitting there waiting for me to make them a cup of tea or coffee. That is one of the things I tell people now — let them do it for you; but I wouldn't have thought of that then. The big things take care of themselves usually, but it is little things that are nice.

Letting others help you — that can be a difficult step to take. For very independent people, it is hard to ask for help, but it is available; it is amazing just what is out there. I had my mastectomy in a small private hospital in the outer eastern suburbs of Melbourne. There were three ladies, including myself, who had mastectomies that week, and we formed our own little group: we called it the Lopsided Ladies Club. Two of us moved away, but we all used to meet quite often, and the nurse who looked after us used to join in. We had a lot of fun; we formed our own little network.

I'm not one for big groups, which is why I like the idea of counselling and helping — because it is one on one.

I have learned so much in all the different things I've done since then, that I probably am different from what I was before. I don't know what's made it happen, but I do feel a lot more confident — game to try different challenges. Having cancer made me think more deeply about different aspects of my life. When you are going through it, everyone says, 'Think positive things,' but you are allowed to have all the other feelings as well. Sometimes I still have a cry under the shower. I find it an easy way if I'm upset about something; people who think at a deep and meaningful level might think you are washing your tears away, but I just found it was a place I could go and you came out and nobody knew you'd been crying. It is hard — you are trying to be positive and strong for your family because everyone has still got their life to live; people still have to go to work, school; you've got to do the housework, the shopping, cook meals. That doesn't all stop because you've got cancer, but if you can get it out of your system somehow — I just found that it was good for me.

Jasmine Reed

Cancer made me stop. For many years I'd probably been doing way too much and not really nurturing my inner self. It made me stop, reflect and then slow down. When you are going through the chemotherapy, you can't do much else but slow down! If it weren't for cancer, I would still be on that same merry-go-round; I don't think anything would have changed.

When Jasmine Reed (not her real name) was diagnosed with breast cancer in 2003, she had started a Master of Neuropsychology, but found that she was more interested in counselling. With her diagnosis her academic plans were put on hold, but she was determined that when she got through her treatments she would use her academic knowledge coupled with her personal life experience to help others. After her treatment, she applied for a place in a Master of Counselling Psychology program, but was refused entry; she was advised that if she died, it would be disruptive to the other students. Jasmine was eventually accepted into a psychology internship program and specialised in trauma therapy. She is now working as a counsellor to women diagnosed with breast cancer. 'Had it not been for my own diagnosis of breast cancer, I would never have ended up where I am,' Jasmine says. 'My life has been enriched in many different ways.'

JASMINE REED: I had a huge psychological base of knowledge in regards to trauma and stress and how they impact on your life. So when I was diagnosed I was able to pull together those theories I'd learned and apply them to myself. Nothing will ever prepare you for those words, 'You have cancer.' It doesn't matter how many books you read, it is very different receiving the diagnosis yourself. But having the background knowledge and the education, I did a lot of writing and a lot of narrative work and a lot of analysis of what was actually happening for me. When I wrote it and analysed it I could say, 'Oh, I get what is going on now.' So it was just a godsend having that degree behind me; it actually helped me through my diagnosis.

At the time I saw [being rejected for the Master of Counselling Psychology program] as a huge negative. I thought, 'Not only have I had to face this potentially life-threatening disease but now I'm really unsure about my academic future as well.' So, for me, it was like a double blow. I thank God that I had some really good people behind me. My surgeon said to me, 'Jasmine, if you can't do things one way, you have to search and find another way.' You know, if she hadn't said those words I would have thought, 'This is the end.' But I was able to say, 'Okay, I can't do what I had proposed to do in the way that I had planned to do it, so I will look at alternatives.' And that is what I did.

Cancer made me stop. For many years I'd probably been doing way too much and not really nurturing my inner self. It made me stop, reflect and then slow down. When you are going through the chemotherapy, you can't do much else but slow down! If it weren't for cancer, I would still be on that same merry-go-round; I don't think anything would have changed. My cancer diagnosis changed it all, and for me, that was a great positive.

I had great support from my immediate family: my husband, my children, my sister and her family, and my brother-in-law and his family. My mum didn't deal well with my diagnosis at all and I accept that now; she couldn't understand why her daughter was diagnosed and why it couldn't have been her. At first I was annoyed with her, angry, as one would be, but when I really broke it down — once again applying psychological knowledge that I had — I realised what was underneath that anger was really just disappointment and sadness. I have a wonderful relationship with my mum now — we always have had a good relationship — she just didn't cope well with my diagnosis.

I had a big group of friends and people who I thought would have been there to support me, but some deserted me, and people who were not so high up in my category of 'good friends' shocked me. I thought, 'Am I such a bad judge of character?' I ran into a girlfriend of mine up at the shops, and when she saw me she walked the other way. She had been one of my very best friends. I'm a little bit confrontational, so I ran after her and said to her, 'Look, what's going on?' and she said, 'Jasmine, I cannot deal with your cancer diagnosis, I don't know how to deal with it.' I guess we are all entitled to feel the way that we feel. A lot of people are scared about cancer. I no longer count her as a friend, because I think friends need to be there not only in good times but in bad times. But I'm not bitter about it; I just say that's how she is. From now on I don't want friends like that, I want friends who are going to be nurturing and supportive in my good times and bad times. Maybe I came to realise these people around me weren't all that I thought they were. Maybe I wasn't all that I thought I was, either; relationships are a two-way street.

[In my counselling work now] I say to women, 'I don't exactly know what you are experiencing,' but sometimes I use a bit of self-disclosure and I say, 'When I was going through my diagnosis, this was the feeling I had.' In a way it gives me more than the textbook knowledge, it gives me greater empathy because I have a shared experience: I've walked their walk, I've talked their talk. I just feel this greater level of connectivity because of that shared experience. You do have certain things that you can't describe to other people unless they have been through it. Someone might talk about their experience of chemotherapy and I'll reflect back and think, 'I remember that feeling,' but I might not say that. Yet I feel that I'm able to reach out to them on a different level.

I work with women in this area in counselling, and death is something that comes up all the time. And, you know what? I'm very comfortable with it: it doesn't scare me, it doesn't faze me. Life is a series of ins and outs: all of us come into the world but some leave earlier than others. I think there is an afterlife and I believe in spirits, so [that belief] I will go on to a different round of experience perhaps. If I was to face a recurrence tomorrow, I don't think that I would be as frightened as I was initially when I was first diagnosed because I've reached a greater sense of where I'm at. I've been able to dwell on those issues of life and death and face my own mortality. I don't want to end up going to my grave angry and bitter; I would rather say, 'This is my life path; this is where it is taking me,' and I would like to think that my life had some purpose in it.

Dr Ian Roos

One of the amazing things this has done for me is put me in a position where I can actually make a difference. That is a real positive when you think about it … It is actually a very privileged position.

Dr Ian Roos is the chair of Cancer Voices Victoria (an advocacy group for those affected by cancer) and a volunteer with the Cancer Council Victoria. He has advanced prostate cancer. That, combined with 20 years' experience in cancer research and his later work in human resource development and adult education, makes him uniquely qualified to influence cancer policy. Cancer has softened him, he says, making him more tolerant of other people's foibles and more compassionate about their problems.

IAN ROOS: Being diagnosed with cancer happened nine years ago. I am not a person who goes to support groups but I did do a bit of a hunt around the internet and found a list server that was very specific for my type of cancer and the type of treatment I was going to have. I subscribed to that and found it really useful: being able to just lurk around the edges of it and see what was happening, to be able to make some comments on specific information as I wanted to and at the times I wanted to — it wasn't something where you had to be there at a specific time or anything like that. It was useful for me, but also it introduced me to two people who were at the same stage of their treatment; we were having our treatment days apart, so we could swap stories of our experiences: one in California, one in Sydney and myself in Melbourne. Because I found that so useful, I contacted the Cancer Council Victoria to say, 'Look, it would be really great if something like this was available in Australia.' The one I belonged to was North American-based and while very helpful, an awful lot of their material reflected their health-care system rather than the Australian one.

At the time I got in touch with the Cancer Council, they were setting up Cancer Connect. They recruited five men who had prostate cancer and asked me to come along to their first meeting and first training day. I was a lecturer in an educational faculty, concentrating on training and development in industry, so the Cancer Council said, 'You can help us in that capacity; tell us about our training and how we can improve it.' So I did that, and then they turned around and said to me, 'Look, you don't meet our requirements as a volunteer but we'd like you to be one because we don't have anyone else who has had your particular treatment.' So they enrolled me in Cancer Connect, and the rest, as you might say, is history.

I was asked to help set up Cancer Voices Victoria, and one of the things we wanted to do was survey people who had cancer to find out what their needs were, what we could address. We had somebody on the committee who had experience in this area, so he sat down and mapped out a survey and we ran it past the committee. One of the comments, from a young lady, was, 'You are just asking people about the negative experience they have; you haven't heard any positive experiences.' His response was, 'Well, I haven't had any.' Immediately just about everybody else said, 'Yes, but we have.' They were talking about changes in attitudes, all those sorts of things. So it was interesting: here was a group of people saying look, despite all the negatives, there are positives.

Obviously, nobody wants to get cancer. I have had a fairly good journey; I haven't had a lot of bad things happen in my journey. Yes, it has left me with some problems and it is still ongoing — I haven't got rid of the cancer. But on a deeply personal level, it has made me a lot more tolerant regarding other people — other people's foibles, other people's problems. I used to say that I don't suffer fools gladly; I wouldn't say that now.

Cancer is the first challenge to your mortality; you want to try to make meaning out of what's happened to you, and in doing that it also changes who you are. I am still essentially the same person, but I would like to think that some of the rougher edges have been knocked off me. I've got a son who gave us a really hard time when he was a teenager; he's got quite a few problems, he is now on a disability support pension. A couple of years ago he turned around to me and said, 'Dad, you've changed.' He didn't need to say more, I knew what he was talking about. I had become a lot more patient with him, a lot more tolerant of some of the silly things he gets up to without thinking, a lot more tolerant of his condition.

I remember being involved in a study of 17 men who had experienced prostate cancer. As I was interviewing them, that aspect of change and increased tolerance was something that was common. Some of them would deny that they'd changed, and then they'd detail all the areas where they had changed. Increased tolerance was a common element. I've got on tape one person saying, 'There is somebody I work with. Once upon a time I would say, "You are a real turkey; I can't be bothered working with you." Now I'll sit down and I'll work with them and try to understand where they are coming from.'

There always was a spiritual dimension for me: I was an active churchgoer and I had a fairly deep faith beforehand. I suspect working with a whole lot of people in the cancer area is a new way of expressing that. I also think it has heightened my sense of social justice; I don't know quite why — I think I am much more socially aware than I was beforehand.

One of the other big positives from cancer is that it has introduced me to some absolutely wonderful people. It's given me a new list of people I now value as friends who I wouldn't have met if this hadn't occurred to me. I would include among my friends now my radiation oncologist, people in the health system … I've just walked across the road and got a big hug and kiss from a lady who is in the Cancer Council Australia who I would never have met beforehand. It is absolutely fascinating — there are so many dedicated people.

One of the amazing things cancer has done for me is put me in a position where I can actually make a difference. That is a real positive when you think about it. For 20 years I was a biomedical researcher in the cancer area; I was involved in the development of anti-cancer drugs. I then moved out of that: I got an invitation to run one of the Melbourne university residential colleges. I did that for five-and-a-half years while I retrained myself as a social scientist and moved into the Graduate School of Management and then an educational faculty. That combination of cancer and scientific know-how and social science, plus the fact I've had cancer, puts me in a fairly unique position at a time when governments are rewriting their cancer policies. It is actually a very privileged position.

I have on my wall a quote from Tim Costello: 'There are times in life when we have to face the big questions, to look squarely into the face of death and then affirm the sheer gift of life.' That really resonates with me. You confront your mortality — by all the statistics I shouldn't be here, but I am and I am very grateful for that, and it puts a new meaning to life.

Professor Glenn Marshall

One of the things that keeps me going every day is the amazing energy — emotional or physical — that parents have. They will do almost anything to make sure their child gets the best possible care ... It is fantastic to work with parents who take that view.

Professor Glenn Marshall is a paediatric haematologist and oncologist, Director of the Centre for Children's Cancer and Blood Disorders at the Sydney Children's Hospital, Randwick. He has worked in treating children with cancer for more than 20 years. He is also head of the Molecular Carcinogenesis Program at the Children's Cancer Institute Australia. Professor Marshall describes profound life changes in the families he deals with and in the adolescents who grow up fast through cancer — and the positive impacts on him and for his staff, despite the tolls of working with young cancer patients.

GLENN MARSHALL: There are lots of ways these experiences positively affect people, the simplest being that the triumph over adversity of having a life-threatening illness changes the parents and siblings. One very common thing said by children who have been cured of a cancer — particularly in their adolescent years — and are getting back in the normal world is that they have grown as people into young adults:

they have matured quickly through having to face and successfully beat the cancer.

One of the things that keeps me going every day is the amazing energy, emotional or physical, that parents have. They will do almost anything to make sure their child gets the best possible care — and hopefully a cure for their disease — and that the side effects of the treatment are minimal. It is fantastic to work with parents who take that view. Some people say there is a high divorce rate in couples who have children with cancer, but that is not my experience at all. You see some who divorce, but for those who stay together, their bond is often stronger. And those that stay together are stronger in their views of what is important in the world; perhaps less acquisitional and less focused on the material things and a bit more focused on the joys of the emotional growth of the child.

I think some people are 'glass half-full', and others 'glass half-empty', so it depends on what sort of person you are as to how you roll with the punches. Most people say to me they expect the worst and hope for the best. We try to understand who these people are and we become their friend and confidant in a way — or at least someone they trust — and work with the individual personality of the parents to help them try to get through it.

As a professional you have to learn who you are dealing with first, and it is best not to go in with too many [fixed] impressions. I try to treat all families or carers in the same way at the outset and try to learn what works for them. Earning their trust is the most important aspect of what we do, and then catering to their emotional and individual needs as time goes on. Going through the experience of cancer treatment can bring out some strengths they may not have thought to exist — and also some instabilities. We do have problem families, and by and large they are people who have extreme problems before we meet them — but you are really talking extremes, not most people.

There is certainly an enormous difference between the experience for a child of seven and a child of 15. The child at 15 has many more changes happening in their life; they are just beginning to engage in the world. Suddenly they lose their hair, they look different; suddenly they are missing chunks of school and social contacts. That is terrible for them. A 15-year-old will have difficulty in relating to other 15-year-olds who have not had to face death, so they often find talking to older adults easier than talking about who is wearing what, or what the latest music is. That pales into insignificance compared with what is important — whether you are going to die the next day. So when they finish their treatment there is a struggle with getting back into normal things with kids their own age. They really are very vulnerable and need long-term psychological and emotional help — probably much more so than your child of seven, eight or nine. Most of the younger kids don't remember much.

We do support parents in a lot of ways. We have a parent support group which consists of parents who have had some training in counselling other parents whose child had cancer. They meet regularly, and the program is co-ordinated by the hospital's social work staff. You discover that people find each other somehow — they meet someone in the ward who says, 'You should talk to so and so.' Then what happens is a small group of people who come from different country areas try to come down on the same date, when their kids are coming for scans or X-rays to make sure the cancer is not coming back. Because they spend the whole weekend at the hospital, they do things around town and keep in touch that way. So there is often a very strong and very positive bond with families who experience this hardship.

I often get parents to try to write things down, how they got through it, because that helps other parents. I did a clinic in Coffs Harbour recently and one family were telling me their story. Dad went back to their home in a regional area and Mum stayed at the hospital for months and months. Now they are back home and their story is about keeping the normal things going. For the dad, working the 12- or 14-hour days may not be as important now as spending time with the family [so he might opt for a less pressured], lower-paid job. What they are seeking is normalisation of life as a family. They realise the stresses and strains of normal adult life are not justifiable in the face of a near-death experience.

Tania Menzies

I was overwhelmed by the volunteers who wanted to help — they all had wonderful qualifications, and most of them had had cancer themselves or in their family. Most of the nannies now on the [community nanny] program have been touched by cancer ... They all think of the program as some way to give back, and to support and help people through hard times in their lives.

Owner of Jelli Beanz Babysitters, Tania Menzies decided to set up a community nanny program for cancer patients after her godmother, Donna Goudie (see page 115), described to her the challenges facing women going through chemo who had young children. Still only in her early 20s, Tania is an energetic person who tackles challenges head-on; she was determined to make something positive happen from Donna's illness. 'Donna is more like a mum, a best friend or a soul mate than a godmother to me,' Tania says. 'The challenge of knowing that your best friend has a terminal illness has brought something amazing for me.'

TANIA MENZIES: I went down to Melbourne in July 2007 to open a branch of Jelli Beanz. Donna was going to be my manager in the Melbourne branch; then while I was down there, she went out of remission. One day, she came home from chemo, she went into her room and took her medication, then came back and said she had a good idea.

Donna is full of good ideas, so I waited for it. She said she thought they needed some program for volunteers to help people going through chemotherapy. Her friend had a baby and was going through chemo, and she was talking about how difficult it was to find childcare and how expensive and how hard it was to find someone you could trust. Donna had the idea of a volunteer organisation run by the local council. I came back to Sydney and thought a bit about it; I emailed a few newspapers to say that I had a volunteer organisation and that I was giving care with my nannies for women with cancer, to see how I could promote my service. I didn't know how I would find families or nannies. Within three days, a newspaper got back to me saying it was a great story, could they come and take photographs and could I tell them more information. So I stayed up very late writing programs, policies and procedures; I contacted all my nannies; I put ads up for volunteers at Sydney Uni and other places.

That's how the program was born. I emailed the NSW Cancer Council and told them how much progress I had made: I emailed several hundred times to different email addresses on their website. Finally they called me and asked me to come and meet with them. I approached the council with the training package and said that I couldn't do this myself because I didn't have the skills as a trainer. I believed then it was going to be a volunteer organisation and I didn't at that stage have best practice for a volunteer organisation — you have to have sufficient training and insurance. So I asked, 'Could the Cancer Council find training and insurance for me and I'll do everything else?' — I'd organise it, I'd get volunteers and I'd get sponsorship so it wouldn't cost them anything — I didn't want to burden their resources. They said they were more than happy to fund all my admin for the first six months. Our program launched on 16 November 2007 with 25 volunteers, working in conjunction with RPA [Royal Prince Alfred Hospital] and we are able to give women unlimited care. Going forward, it is not going to be volunteers; we will offer paid nannies — the Cancer Council is funding it. We are hoping after a six-month trial we can launch it throughout Australia.

At the time this book went to press, a year after this interview, the program involved 12 full-time nannies working with oncology units at every hospital in Sydney, and was continuing to grow.

I was overwhelmed by the volunteers who wanted to help — they all had wonderful qualifications, and most of them had had cancer themselves or in their family. Most of the nannies now on the [community nanny] program have been touched by cancer. We decided that if they'd gone through their own cancer experience in the last two years to wait and maybe have them as a volunteer on our weekend program, just because we want to look after their mental health and make sure they are coping with it. This morning I was looking through my enrolment forms and out of 25 nannies, only four of them haven't had some kind of experience with cancer, whether it be their grandparents or friends — so that is kind of shocking as well. They all think of the program as some way to give back, and to support and help people through hard times in their lives.

It just makes so much sense to have a nanny agency with qualified people who want to offer this kind of help. That is what their motivation is: they work with children because they love children. Why not then help someone who really needs it, rather than trying to focus on finding clients who already have amazing care they can afford to pay for? I want to pitch the program to individuals who couldn't afford the best people, so that they can have the best care for their children.

Lee Murphy

You start to value every moment. You decide not to put off doing the things that press your buttons, make you happy, fulfil your dreams, stir your passion. You live a little more boldly and bravely, and it seems like you don't have so much to lose in trying those things.

After suffering from chronic fatigue syndrome for 15 years, Lee Murphy faced a diagnosis of breast cancer in 2007. Her first feeling was annoyance — in her busy life, cancer was an extraordinarily inconvenient intrusion. Her next thought was, 'I can do this, I've been here before.' Lee deals with cancer with a lavish dose of irreverent (some would say morbid) humour —

even when she is planning her own funeral. A singer and a songwriter, since her diagnosis Lee has also found enormous solace and fresh inspiration in her music.

LEE MURPHY: I couldn't stand intense, pitying or morbid responses. I think because I'm so 'out there' about [having cancer], people are quite shocked. I'll make a joke about nipples or something and people tentatively relax and laugh. They say something like, 'You seem really positive about it!' — they're surprised. I don't know if I don't take it seriously enough or if that's just how I deal with it … It is almost like I am a bit disrespectful about cancer.

Waiting for my diagnosis took five excruciating weeks. In that time you process all your worst fears regarding what might happen to you — including the very real possibility of death. One night during those weeks, I had been sobbing while playing a Tori Amos song over and over, when I decided I'd like it played at my funeral. I knew it was morbid but I told my girlfriend Tracy, who had cancer some years ago, 'I started planning my funeral,' waiting to be told off for being negative. But her response was, 'I did the same thing.' I felt relieved that maybe it was normal, given the circumstances. Trace is an actress with a great sense of drama and humour and so we got on a bit of a roll about our respective funeral plans. I felt I should write my own songs and record them for the occasion — with friends and family saying, 'Just can't shut her up; she's still singing from the grave.' Tracy and I are both a little 'anal retentive' about being organised — she'd planned to accessorise herself in her favourite pink to match the casket lining. We decided that before we left, we would have written the orders of service and our own eulogies, designed our booklets, flower arrangements and food for the wake — everything down to the last detail, leaving nothing to chance or to lesser planners than ourselves. As I wanted to be cremated, we decided I was going to wear something highly flammable; she allocated me beige polyester and some Homy Peds — it seemed I wasn't going out looking cool! … It was all highly distasteful, and we didn't mean any disrespect, but when you look death squarely in the face, what are you supposed to do or say — we decided to laugh! Those plans are on the backburner for now — we're not planning to die any time soon.

Cancer is like an evil word, a feared word. When I was diagnosed, I'd been through the ringer, because for two years I'd been pretty much housebound [with chronic fatigue syndrome]. They were just terrible times; some days I felt I'd rather put a bullet in my head if this was how I was going to be forever. I couldn't function, I couldn't think, I could hardly move, even to do the basic things. It was literally a struggle to survive. So when I was diagnosed I thought, 'Here we go, I have to dig deep again. I can do this, I've been here before.' I was annoyed: I had just got back on my feet, I was developing my property, I'd just landscaped my garden and I thought, 'I have not got time for cancer.' It was extraordinarily inconvenient … it could be a whole year of surgery, chemo and treatments. It was extremely intrusive in my life, so I was really pissed off.

Overall I've felt carried by the people close to me; it is like many strong arms have carried me through. I think it would be really hard not to have had that, and I probably reached a point of acceptance about receiving help and having to ask for it. I learned that through my last illness; I'm normally very self-sufficient, brought up not to rely on anyone else. But by the time I got cancer, I was willing and able to receive, and people have been mostly supportive. It scares some people: it gives them a bit of a wake-up call, perhaps about how they treated you before or the status of your relationship with them. A friend I hadn't heard from for some time found out I had cancer and sent an email the week before my nine-hour surgery, wanting to resolve our relationship issues. I replied, 'It's really not the time to be dealing with this — thanks, I'll get back to you later.' My ex-husband suddenly became very attentive and helpful, and seemed to reach some personal crisis point. I'd been sick for 15 years with another illness — diabolically so for two years — but cancer seems to alarm people.

Some people got very teary and emotional and intense about it, and I could not handle that at all; I needed a light positive approach. I've had my moments where I'll cry and feel lost, but I can't handle that response. On the whole, I like it when people are natural about it, when they listen to my fears or help me go through the process of making decisions.

My life might now be a bit shorter, but none of us really knows. The thought struck me, 'Okay, what if I have, say, five years to live? How do I really want to spend those days and years and who do I want to spend them with?' You start to value every moment. You decide not to put off doing the things that press your buttons, make you happy, fulfil your dreams, stir your passion. You live a little more boldly and bravely, and it seems like you don't have so much to lose in trying those things. Suddenly, trying to work and save for a secure, happier retirement seems less important than living for today. It's that whole *Sliding Doors* thing: I might sell my house, go to Tuscany, become an artist, sell a whole lot of paintings — have a whole different life. But only if I dare to take the risk — something that would have seemed irresponsible to me before, when I lived more fearfully. Sometimes risks pay off in ways we never dreamed of. We just can't see what might come from taking a step off the planned path.

I asked myself, 'If you could do anything, what would it be?' My answer was, 'To sing and play with other musicians.' I've been doing it all my life, to varying degrees, but I wanted to go professional. This year, just prior to the cancer and since, I've been prolific with my songwriting. I've been meeting many talented musicians and singers — it's been amazing. Doors have been opening for me to step through. Songwriting tends to be a bit of therapy, like a journal: I can process my life through what I write, and sometimes it helps formulate what I am experiencing. Songs have to be so succinct; you only have four minutes to catch the whole theme, so it does make you think about the subject you are trying to write about.

I studied business admin and thought I could get a part-time job to fit in with my CFS, but that is not a passion, it is a way to pay the bills. Music is what I love — and if I can make money doing it, that's great. I've been asked to do a lot of things with music in the past that I've had to turn down because of family life and commitments. I have to do something to make a living, make a choice to go in one direction, so while I've got the freedom to do it now, I will see where it leads me and I won't die wondering, 'What if?'

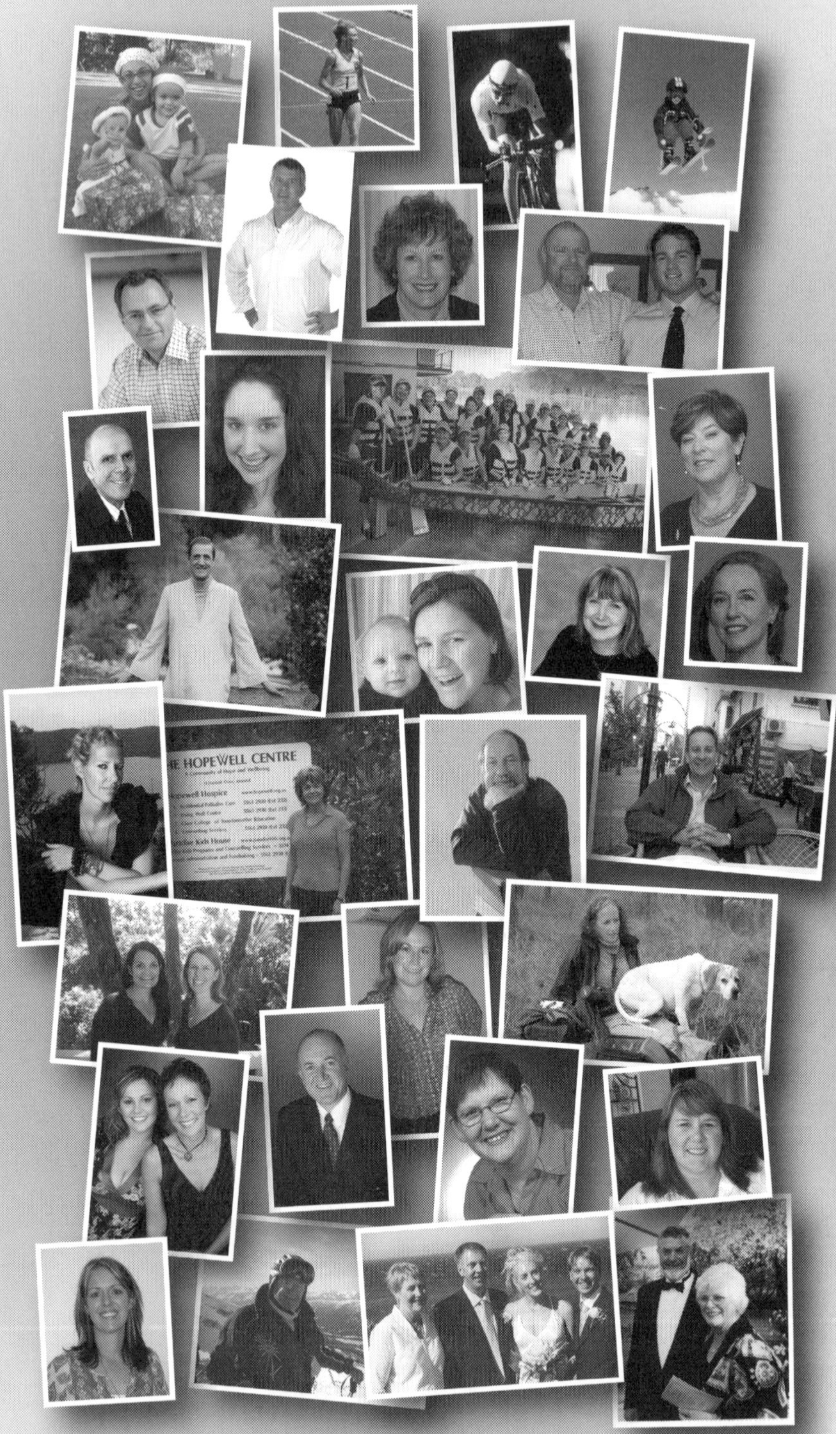
HOPEWELL CENTRE

CHAPTER 6

Turning back the clock

> Time is but the stream I go a-fishing in. I drink at it; but while I drink, I see the sandy bottom and detect how shallow it is. Its thin current slides away, but eternity remains. I would drink deeper; fish fill the sky, whose bottom is pebbly with stars. I cannot count one. I know not the first letter of the alphabet. I have always been regretting that I was not as wise as the day I was born.
>
> **Henry David Thoreau (1817–62)**

'If you could turn back the clock and take cancer out of the equation, would you do it?'

It seems like the most obvious question in the world, hardly worth asking. But I asked it in almost every interview for this book, and some of the answers were surprising. The responses were rarely black and white — yes or no — which brings home what an intricate blend of blessing and burden cancer can be.

Deirdre Hanna

BREAST CANCER

I don't think that I would. I can't say what specifically would stop me doing that, other than I think it is part of my journey. I think I needed to have this experience, and I'd rather have it now than when I'm in my 80s or 90s, when I might still have the same fears but maybe not the same group of support people around me. I've got just the most amazing group of family, friends and medical team, and that's made an incredible difference. I wasn't alone at any stage. I tend to isolate myself a bit, I'm a bit of a loner and a bit of an introvert — I know it doesn't sound like that! — but accepting help was big because I'm very independent. I was given every opportunity emotionally through my friends and support group, and physically through the evolution of medicine and through the most noble team of men in charge of my surgery, reconstruction and oncology — I've never been really trusting of male doctors and I probably got three of the best. I was really fortunate, so I think, 'How can I change something that was so positive?'

Raelene Boyle

BREAST CANCER AND OVARIAN CANCER

Obviously, if you were not diagnosed with cancer, you wouldn't choose it! But it has given me great opportunities to meet wonderful people who are inspirational and don't deserve what they've been struck with. I've also met amazingly committed surgeons, researchers and doctors who make a massive difference in our community. And I've ended up living here in Buderim on the Sunshine Coast, moving away from a city — all those decisions I probably wouldn't have been able to make without this life crisis. Cancer gave me the credentials to be able to make difficult decisions.

Chris Reason

PROSTATE CANCER

It would be stupid of me to say everybody should go through it to teach themselves these lessons ... You'd like to think that there is some way of learning other than having to go through it yourself. I wish I had never had to go through it; it was horrific and it was difficult and it was exceedingly painful and a very low time in my life. But I look at the overwhelming positives that came out of it and the life-changing experiences and lessons that I got from it. Could I have got those any other way? No. Would I have the perspective I have on life now without having gone through that? No. So it was the only way that I would have come to the point that I'm at in my life now. It makes me appreciate my wife so much more, my kids so much more and my life so much more. I could never have learned that from reading your book, or watching a TV interview, or talking to a cancer survivor. The lessons you learn in that cancer classroom are exclusive. It is a special club, and I'm honoured to have graduated — but I don't know if I'd ever enrol again.

Lyndie Powell

SON, NICHOLAS, HAD STAGE 4 NEUROBLASTOMA

Absolutely, there is nothing worse. It is lovely to have the ski trips [Nicholas competes in skiing events for transplant recipients] but to have a healthy child and not have to go through everything we have? — no question about it.

Tali Foreman & Karen Johnston

SYDNEY CHILDREN'S HOSPITAL

TALI: Yes, definitely. All the positive effects or outcomes will never outweigh the cancer itself and the damage it can do. I think every single person who works in this unit would want a magic wand to wish it away. Because there are also the people who don't get to experience the positive effects.

KAREN: If you ever find that wand, I'm sure we could find other jobs …

Tess Berthelson

OVARIAN CANCER

Yes, I would, I think. I wouldn't want [cancer] even though there have been changes; I don't consider my life was less rich before. One main reason for changing the 'cancer' diagnosis, if I could, is that I hate to see the current suffering of my family and to know that there may be a lot more to come. Of course I would change that if I could.

Dr Ian Gawler

BONE CANCER

I am not sure that particular question is a helpful one to even fantasise about. There is no doubt it would be much nicer if I had learned all this stuff and still had two legs and not gone through some of the difficulty I did 30 years ago, but the reality is that is not what happened.

Michael Barnes

PROSTATE CANCER

This is not very clear-cut, but yes and no. The 'yes' is about discovering a partner who will travel through that stuff with me, which is pretty special. It is entirely hypothetical to try to figure out what might have happened to us if I hadn't [had cancer], but I do really appreciate her love and support during that time. The 'no' is that cancer is just crap. I am very wary of people who sentimentalise these things — I just don't think it is true to the ambiguity and complexity of life.

Celeste Powell

HODGKIN'S LYMPHOMA

Definitely not. It is not all positive of course, it can't be, but I don't think today I would take back the whole experience, even the negatives. It sounds clichéd, but cancer has shaped me to be who I am today. I've met people that I wouldn't have otherwise, and I've got a greater understanding of the more important things in life. It has changed my whole outlook into a positive one, and I have a more mature approach to things, which is something that I wouldn't have, had it not been for my illness.

Diana Davidson

BREAST CANCER AND ADVANCED SECONDARY CANCERS

At this stage of my life I wouldn't turn anything away; it has all been part of the pattern. You have to learn acceptance. I do say the prayer, 'God grant me the serenity to accept the things I cannot change, courage to change the things I can and wisdom to know the difference.' When an event has gone past, all the wisdom in the world is not going to take the time back.

Heidi Middleton

BREAST CANCER

Most definitely. Even though I feel richer and stronger, it is still something you wouldn't wish on your worst enemy. There are amazing and wonderful things that come out of the experience, but you still wouldn't wish it upon someone. So most definitely; I really pray for a cure in my daughter's lifetime. It does still take lives, it is a killer. You never ever believe it is going to enter your realm, but it does.

Liz Stone & Sharon Tregoning

BREAST CANCER AND ADVANCED SECONDARY CANCERS (LIZ)

LIZ: No, no. And I always said if I was offered something to change my daughter [who has a genetic disability], I wouldn't take that, either; her disability is intrinsically part of who she is.

SHARON: Yes and no. Cancer has certainly been the catalyst for our relationship and given how much I treasure it, I wouldn't want to mess with that. From the perspective that I'm not going to have Liz around for a long time — yes, without a second thought.

Mike Schram

WIFE, ELAINE, DIED OF OVARIAN CANCER

No. I would have to set Elaine aside and say it was something I had to go through. I wouldn't change anything in my life at all anyway, because I do think that things happen to you for a reason and — it sounds trashy — they make you a better person for the good of the general picture. My way of looking at it was, her job was done. I'm not happy that I don't have somebody to cuddle in the morning, but she accomplished an awful lot. If she's not on her next assignment, she will have one — I do think there is continuance that way.

Claire Harrop

MOTHER DIED OF CERVICAL CANCER, SON ANGUS DIED FROM A BRAIN TUMOUR

I would say yes, because I would want my family back; on the other hand, I wouldn't know what I know and I wouldn't have the feelings that I have now. I wasn't a very compassionate person before. But I would definitely want my family back.

Deena Raphael

MOTHER DIED OF CANCER

I would give anything to have [my mother] here, but also I am a big believer in the domino effect. I left [the US] to travel the world for just a year or two; that was 12 years ago. Since then I've lived in Vietnam, met my husband, moved to Australia and had two kids. And my stepmother — my dad isn't married to her now, but they were married for about nine years — is a really strong person in my life. So all those things would never have happened if my mother hadn't died, which is so tragic, but for me there are so many things that are positive. This is what my life is and that is how it has played out, and I just try to go with the flow.

Lauren Adlam

MOTHER DIED OF CANCER

Absolutely, if I could turn back time and cure cancer the year before [my mother] was diagnosed — I'd make a fortune, too! If we knew the end result was always going to be the same, the way it happened was probably a good way. It was a relatively short amount of time she was suffering, so from that point of view, the way it happened was quite good. But if I could change it, I would in a heartbeat.

Karen Forster

BREAST CANCER; HUSBAND DANNY DIED OF PARANASAL SINUS CANCER

No, certainly my own I wouldn't, because I think it was meant to happen to me. I needed something, some bolt of lightning, to say, 'Take a look at yourself: where are you going and what are you doing?' There are parts of my husband's cancer that I would like to take away: the nasty parts, the pain, the suffering. It was bloody awful; there was no two ways about it. It went into his brain and ate away at his skull; the mechanics of it were just awful, and I'd like to take that away. But it was in lots of ways a gift to know he was dying. We didn't know when but we knew it was going to be some time, so [it was a chance] to do the things you wanted to do, to say the things you wanted to say. It is a precious gift to be given that tap on the shoulder to say, 'Don't wait.'

Lyn Swinburne

BREAST CANCER

No, no, I wouldn't take it away, because for me it has been a chance to discover a lot of things about myself, to unearth talents and skills and insights that would not have shown themselves otherwise.

Sally Crossing

BREAST CANCER

Oh, yes. [Without cancer] I don't know what I'd be doing right now; I might be doing something even more rewarding and fascinating, but in the latter part of life, it has given me an unexpectedly satisfying purpose and career — definitely more satisfying than the one I had before. The combination of giving back and being able to make things change for the better is very heady stuff.

Dr Ian Roos

ADVANCED PROSTATE CANCER

Yes, no doubt about that. When you look at the effect of cancer on the individuals, their families and those who love them, then there is only one answer to that.

Lisa Humphreys

MOTHER DIED OF BREAST CANCER

My instinct says of course I would take it away. I would love my mother back and every day I want my life with her back. But on the other hand, I would not be the person I am today if it wasn't for [cancer]; I wouldn't have the relationship I have with my brother and I probably wouldn't have the relationship I have with my father — because that dramatically changed over the time she was ill. My parents were divorced when I was 12. When Mum passed away, I think my father had this amazing light go on in his head. For him it was a big wake-up call — he suddenly realised he didn't have a very close relationship with his children. He started taking more interest in our lives, and we became a lot closer. The same with my grandparents. As time went on, we got a lot closer. They were my mum's parents, and as I matured I suddenly realised, 'My God, these people gave birth to my amazing mother; there is something amazing in them as well.' That relationship is just so special now. And my relationship with my brother: people can't believe how close we are. We cared for my mother together; we became each other's life. Before, my brother and I fought a lot — we just didn't have that deeper connection that we have now, so that is something I would never want to go back and miss out on.

Lee Murphy

BREAST CANCER

I don't know if anyone would choose to have cancer. For the rest of my life there is now a question in my mind — will I get it again? Is it somewhere else? What will be the side effects of my medication? Should I remove my ovaries to reduce risk and face early menopause? Will I find a partner despite my scars and my health issues? Cancer does take away a lot, particularly for a young person, but I have gained some positives from it, too. 'Would I have gained them if I didn't get cancer?' is another question. (I probably wouldn't have had the flat tummy!) Maybe cancer was enough to make me take the risk to do what I really wanted to — who knows? It's impossible to know what other paths I might have taken without cancer, to know how much it has impacted on my life and decisions. The biggest lesson I think cancer has taught me is that life really is short, and we need to live it purposefully, intentionally and fully every day of our lives — no matter how long we have on this planet. Today could be the last day for any one of us — I don't want to waste it!

Jason Garrick

FATHER DIED OF METASTATIC MELANOMA

You don't even have to finish that question. The answer is no, I wouldn't change it. Yes, there are times where I'd love [my father] to be here, but he's not — you can't change that. I would have loved him to be at my graduation, at my 21st, but the fact of the matter is he isn't. Even if he was, then it would be, 'I wish he was here for this and here for that,' and then that's getting to that victim thing — 'Oh, poor me, he's not here.' I wouldn't change it at all. It happened, and I wouldn't be the person I am now if it didn't happen; my family wouldn't be the way we are now. Even though Dad is not with us any more, he is still living as part of us. He has two sons, myself and Joel, he had a 27-year relationship with Mum and that's still there; the love is still there.

Jasmine Reed

BREAST CANCER

No. As traumatic as the experience was for me, it has been part of my life journey and it has led me to a very serene place. I always had good relationships with my own family; I don't think they are any better, but they are stronger. I would not be working in the position that I'm currently in had it not been for my cancer diagnosis. By the same token, I don't wish for a recurrence, don't get me wrong, but if it happens, it happens — I can't change that but I'll do whatever I can to get myself well again, if that is at all possible.

I'm really happy with where I have got to in my life. As for the future, I don't really project into the future. I find personally that is a dangerous psychological place for me to be; that can lead me into, 'Will I see my children grow up?' Yes, I do want to see my children grow up; I'd love to see them have children, if that is what they choose to do, but I don't project too far into the future. It is just day to day, right here, right now.

Mohamed Khadra

THYROID CANCER

Remove cancer as an eventuality? I must say it's something I've thought of a lot. There are great benefits that have arisen in my life from having to confront cancer. I'm not sure that it's only cancer that does that: people who are stranded on Mount Everest and survive have the same notions. Being brought face to face with your own mortality in any shape or form — this life is a finite commodity and once you are mindful of mortality then you are able to make the best of this life. But would I take cancer out? I'd rather not have gone through the discomfort of those years, but it has certainly brought an enormous amount of growing up to me that I would never have done without cancer. The benefits have been so huge, but I think it's not the cancer itself, it is the growing up you've done as a result of cancer. The fact you had to have cancer before you grew up is, in itself, stupid — why couldn't we grow up without it? A different question is, 'Would I wish for cancer?' The answer to that is no.

Bernadette Martin

HODGKIN'S LYMPHOMA

I probably wouldn't because I think it's made a big difference to my life, but I wish I could have had the knowledge I have now at the start of the treatment. They say you don't appreciate something until you lose it — to nearly lose life made me appreciate life and all of the wonderful people I have in mine. I would rather that I only live another two or five years in a life filled with love and happiness than endure another 50 years of mere existence, which is what I may have done had I not had cancer.

Pauline Welch

BREAST CANCER

I don't know. It was a horrible experience to go through, and you are worried whether or not you are going to come out of it, how you are going to come out of it. But — how do I say this? — I would wish away the disease but maybe not the experience.

Donna Goudie

OVARIAN CANCER

I don't think I'd be brave enough to want *this* cancer. I wouldn't mind a less nasty cancer; some cancers like bowel or breast, you have a lot more chance. This cancer, it seems to be you've got no chance. But then I figure I never do things by halves; if my back wasn't against the wall there is absolutely no way I would have done this work. I was in a dilemma before this: I hated my job for years, but like a lot of people, I spent a lot of time studying to get degrees so I could do it. But the [IT] industry changed and it became much more cut-throat. I felt like I threatened my being every day I went to work; I was so miserable, but I earned a lot of money and I was good at what I did, so I felt like I had no choice. I had to put one foot in front of the other, buy investment properties, become an aspirational Australian — it was like it was all mapped out. One of the first things I did on my healing process was that I said to my husband, Mark, 'I am never going back to IT. I hate it, I've hated it for years. I am not hurting myself like that any more.' I was 46, 47 and I felt like my life was over; all the fun stuff had happened when I was young, now it was just the dregs. I hadn't done anything that I would have loved to have done. Now I've got my freedom. At a terrible price, but cancer has bought my freedom.

Simon O'Donnell

NON-HODGKIN'S LYMPHOMA

No, no. I would never want to not have that knowledge, that experience. I hope with the experience I can help others; I have a great quality of life, I can talk positively about something that will reach in and rip your heart out. So I wouldn't change anything.

Tracey Gaudry

ACUTE LYMPHATIC LEUKAEMIA

Who knows what life would be like if I hadn't had cancer? You wouldn't wish it upon your worst enemy, let alone yourself, but I also say stuff happens for a reason. I was one of the fortunate ones who got through on a shocking prognosis; it gave me qualities which I wouldn't have had otherwise. It is better that I had cancer and got through than someone else have it and not get through. During my treatment I met a young girl, also about 20, with Hodgkin's disease and I would go and visit her in hospital. She didn't go into remission as easily as I did. I remember one day she said, 'I just want to die, it is too hard. I don't want to try any more.' The hardest thing was I couldn't give her even one per cent of my will; I couldn't give her one per cent of my strength; I couldn't give her an ounce of anything I had to help her get through. She passed away less than a week later and that was probably the most difficult part. What was it about me that made me different? Why couldn't she just have some part of it? Make me a little bit sicker so she could be a bit better — I would gladly have been a lot sicker to let someone else live.

I have a hugely fulfilling life with a devoted husband and three beautiful young children. This was definitely not a scene in the picture painted by my medical team when I was 20. In all likelihood the combination, intensity and duration of chemotherapy treatments should have rendered me infertile. What's to want to retract any part of my life?

Stephanie Dowrick

BREAST CANCER; MOTHER DIED OF CANCER

Yes, absolutely. And if I could turn the clock forward, also! I don't want more illness — we have had so much of it in our family. I didn't need cancer to teach me who and what I value. I don't need anyone around me to be ill to teach me how much I love them. No. No. In the face of that awful time — and many other tough times also — I did eventually do my best with it. And I deeply value the book that came out of it (*Forgiveness & Other Acts of Love*). But please believe me: I would like to have avoided all those experiences of utter desolation no matter what the eventual rewards. I am absolutely aware that many people feel in retrospect that what they learned was invaluable. My grandparents outlived four of their seven adult children, so perhaps because death touched my life so early, I already knew more than enough about mortality and grief. My challenge has been to learn more about joy, life, and *this* great moment of living.

Acknowledgments

So many people are a part of this book — not only those whose stories appear here, but others who put me in touch with someone with a tale to tell. For their enthusiasm and passionate support for the concept of *Positive*, I thank the following (and apologise to anyone I've left out):

Sue Brockhoff, Ian and Bette Collings, Michele Corin, Poppy Diamantis and Kylie Rafferty (Sydney Children's Hospital), Jodie Gacitua (CanTeen), Nicci Hunter (Sass & Bide), Belinda Jackson, Carolyn Martin, Lisa Portman and Belinda Goldfinch (Cancer Council Victoria), Russell Powell, Simon Ralph, Angela Rossmanith, Dominic Steele, Georgia Stynes (Cancer Council New South Wales), Rachel Symes, and Katie Thirkhill.

Thanks, too, to the behind-the scenes team: my friends and family in Brisbane, Sydney and Geelong; Janette Doolan, transcriber extraordinaire; and the spectacular bunch at HarperCollins, in particular Shona Martyn, Amruta Slee and Anne Reilly.

Jason Garrick would like to acknowledge the people who helped him through his journey: David Purcell, Chanelle Harvey, Laura Price, Alex Walls, Erin Georgeson, Elizabeth Smith, Lachlan McPherson, Matt Baartz, Adam Jahnke, Justin Bulwinkel, Shayne Fry and Kieren McGuire.

Text permissions

For giving permission to reproduce material in this book, the author and publisher wish to thank the following:

Page 1: *Australian Story* (ABC TV) for the quote from Aaron McMillan in 'Playing for Time', broadcast on 27 September 2001.

Page 53: reprinted with the permission of Simon & Schuster, Inc. from *The Courage to Start: A Guide to Running for Your Life* by John 'The Penguin' Bingham. Copyright © 1999 by John Bingham.

Page 93: reprinted with the permission of Blake Friedmann Literary, TV and Film Agency Ltd from M. Scott Peck, *The Road Less Travelled* (Arrow Books, London 1990).

Page 139: from *Bread for the Journey: A Daybook of Wisdom and Faith* by Henri J.M. Nouwen. Copyright © 1997 by Henri J.M. Nouwen. Reprinted by permission of HarperCollins Publishers and Darton, Longman and Todd Ltd.

Photo details

The following people appear in the chapter-opener photos (top to bottom, left to right):

Chapter 1 — Chris Reason, Bernadette Vella, Celeste Powell, Claire Harrop (with Angus), Jason Garrick (with his father), Jane Turner.

Chapter 2 — Tracey Gaudry, Nicholas Powell, Raelene Boyle, Simon O'Donnell, John Stubbs, the Brave Hearts dragon boat team.

Chapter 3 — Ian Gawler, Deirdre Hanna, Stephanie Dowrick, Michael Barnes.

Chapter 4 — Deena Raphael and Lauren Adlam, Sharon Tregoning, Liz Stone, Heidi Middleton, Sandra Kent, Elaine Schram.

Chapter 5 — Colleen McKay, Geoff Whitelaw, Karen Forster (with husband Danny), Ian Roos, Mohamed Khadra, Lyn Swinburne, Sally Crossing, Tania Menzies and Donna Goudie, Pauline Welch.